The Lectin Free Cookbook

Over 200 Proven, Delicious & Easy for Your Instant Pot Electric Pressure Cooker to Heal Your Gut, Lose Weight & Feel Spectacular. 14 Day Action Plan Included.

Author: Michelle Thomas

Copyright 2018 by Michelle Thomas - All rights reserved.

This document by Michelle Thomas, is geared towards providing exact and reliable information in regards to the topic and issue covered. The publication is sold with the idea that the publisher is not required to render accounting, officially permitted, or otherwise, qualified services. If advice is necessary, legal or professional, a practiced individual in the profession should be ordered.

From a Declaration of Principles which was accepted and approved equally by a Committee of the American Bar Association and a Committee of Publishers and Associations.

In no way is it legal to reproduce, duplicate, or transmit any part of this document in either electronic means or in printed format. Recording of this publication is strictly prohibited and any storage of this document is not allowed unless with written permission from the publisher. All rights reserved.

The information provided herein is stated to be truthful and consistent, in that any liability, in terms of inattention or otherwise, by any usage or abuse of any policies, processes, or directions contained within is the solitary and utter responsibility of the recipient reader. Under no circumstances will any legal responsibility or blame be held against the publisher for any reparation, damages, or monetary loss due to the information herein, either directly or indirectly.

The information herein is offered for informational purposes solely, and is universal as so. The presentation of the information is without contract or any type of guarantee assurance.

The trademarks that are used are without any consent, and the publication of the trademark is without permission or backing by the trademark owner. All trademarks and brands within this book are for clarifying purposes only and are the owned by the owners themselves, not affiliated with this document.

Special Bonus

Ready to receive over 600 Delicious & Easy Recipes for FREE?

We want to thank you for purchasing the book and we hope to make your belly happy with the recipes that follow. As a token of our appreciation we have a little gift for you.
We are a team of small but passionate cookbook writers and our mission is to make cooking fun, simple and delicious. Writing recipes gives us a chance to have fun, be creative and let other people know that healthy and delicious food does not have to be complicated nor take hours and hours.

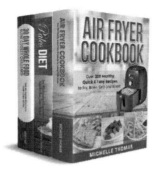

Only sign up for the cookbook box set if you are ready to be absolutely amazed with over 600 proven, delicious and easy to make recipes.

To access the gift page type in www.bit.ly/2Ho82AH or email us at info@limitlessrecipes.com to get the box set delivered to your email.

 Limitless Recipes
Like us on Facebook and join our private Facebook group community for more recipes and gifts.
 @limitlessrecipes
Follow us on Instagram
 Limitless Recipes
Follow us on Pinterest.

Want to be a part of our closed Facebook group?
We are working on building an engaged community discussing recipes and healthy eating in our closed Facebook group. If you would like to be involved in the discussions about cooking, what is working, what is not working and receive information about gifts and promotions, we would be delighted to add you.

Type in Limitless Recipes on Facebook or write us at info@limitlessrecipes.com. Come say hi!

Happy Cooking!

Table of Contents

Introduction 14

    What Exactly Are Lectins & How to Improve Your Relationship with Gluten 14

    The Ultimate Guide to Lectin-Free Life 15

    Top 10 Tips to Stick to The Diet with Ease & Mistakes to Avoid 16

    Your 14 Day Action Plan 18

BREAKFAST 20

    Boiled Eggs 3-Ways 20

    Egg Curry 20

    Tangy Greek-Style Coconut Yogurt 21

    Cheese & Bacon Muffins 21

    Crustless Spinach Quiche 22

    Sweet Potato Hash w/ Mushrooms 22

    Eggs En Cocotte 23

    Tapioca Pearl Pudding 23

    Bacon & Sausage Omelet 24

    Crustless Meaty Quiche 24

    Egg Custard 25

    Ham Casserole 25

    Twice-Baked Sweet Potatoes Casserole 26

    Frosted Egg Frittata Cupcakes 26

    Oef en Cocotte a.k.a French "Baked" Eggs 27

    Scotch Eggs 27

Slow Cooked Ham & Spinach Frittata 28

Sweet Potato Hash 28

Sausage Egg Casserole 29

Slow Cooked Breakfast Chicken Soup 29

Sweet Potato & Collard Hash 30

Breakfast Casserole 30

LUNCH 34

Southwest Chicken w/ Cauliflower Rice 34

Alaska Cod Tacos w/ Lime-Garlic Sour Cream 35

Creamy Chicken Soup 36

One-Pot Pork Belly & Spiced Cauliflower Rice 36

Pear & Almond Chicken Lettuce Wraps 37

Chicken Lettuce Wraps 37

Loaded Beef Stew 38

One-Pot Roast & Sweet Potato-Cauliflower Mash 39

Pulled-Pork Chipotle Salad 39

Lettuce-Wrapped Pulled Pork 40

Zuppa Toscana 41

Turmeric Chicken & Avocado Salad 41

Chicken Taquitos 42

Chicken Shawarma 42

SIDE DISHES 44

2-Ways Cauliflower Rice 44

Steamed Broccoli 44

Caramelized Onions 45

Baked Sweet Potatoes 45

Steamed Asparagus 46

Steamed Carrot Flowers 46

Garlicky Mashed Sweet Potatoes 47

Garlicky Broccoli 47

Steamed Artichokes 48

Brussels Sprouts 48

Cauliflower Mash 49

Saag 49

Turnip Greens & Bacon 50

Cajun Greens 50

Garlic & Lemon Kale 51

Collard Greens & Bacon 51

Braised Kale w/ Carrots 52

Sweet & Sour Red Cabbage 52

Salt & Vinegar Brussel Sprouts 53

Cabbage 53

Cauliflower & Mushroom Risotto 54

Mixed Root Veggie Mash 54

Savoy Cabbage w/ Cream Sauce a.k.a Wirsing mit Sahnesoße) 55

Mashed Sweet Potato Muffin Tin 55

Mashed Sweet Potatoes 56

Carrot & Sweet Potato Mash 57

Sweet Potato & Cauliflower Mash 57

Creamy Cauliflower Risotto 58

Coconut Cabbage 59

Beet Pickles 60

Herbed-Saffron Cauliflower Rice 60

Rustic Root Vegetable Mash 61

SOUPS & STEWS 62

Beef Stew w/ Turnips & Carrots 62

Chicken Soup 62

Sweet Potato & Carrot Soup 63

Italian Soup 63

Beef Meatball Soup 64

Turmeric Sweet Potato Soup 65

Bacon & Potato Chowder 65

Beef Bourguignon 66

Roasted Garlic Sweet Potato Soup 67

Chicken Soup 68

Parmesan, Sweet Potato, & Broccoli Soup 69

Cream of Asparagus Soup 70

No-Noodle Turmeric Chicken Soup 70

Chicken & Bacon Chowder 71

Napa Cabbage & Pork Soup 72

Beef & Broccoli Curry Stew 72

Loaded Cauliflower Soup 73

Fennel & Chicken Soup 73

Hearty Vegetable Soup 74

Beef Stew 74

Sweet Potato & Chorizo Soup 75

Carrot & Leek Turmeric Soup 75

10-Minute Mushroom Broth 76

Carrot & Ginger Soup 76

Chicken & Avocado Soup 77

Balsamic Beef & Cabbage Soup 77

Chicken Vegetable Soup 78

Chicken Drumstick Soup 78

FISH & SEAFOOD 79

Wild Alaskan w/ Broccoli or Cauliflower 79

Steamed Shrimp & Asparagus 79

Crispy Salmon 80

Salmon & Broccoli 80

Clam Chowder 81

Cod Chowder 81

Salmon & Broccoli 82

Pepper-Lemon Salmon 82

10-Minute Salmon 83

Fish & Veggies 83

POULTRY **85**

Chicken & Broccoli Alfredo 85

Creamy Chicken 85

Turkey Breast & Gravy 86

Zuppa Toscana 87

Chicken 2-Ways.. 87

30-Minute Fall-Off-The-Bone Chicken 88

Crack Chicken... 88

Turkey Drumsticks 89

Chicken Wings.. 89

Creamy Chicken & Mushroom 90

Pesto Chicken w/ Carrots & Sweet Potatoes 90

Chicken w/ Sweet Potatoes & Mixed Veggies 91

Turkey & Sweet Potato White Chili... 91

Very Simple Whole Chicken 92

Roasted Whole Chicken 93

Coconut Chicken & Sweet Potato Curry 93

Coconut Basil Chicken Curry 94

Lemon Chicken.. 95

Turkey Breast Roast 95

Chicken Legs W/ Lemon & Garlic 96

Thai Chicken	96
Lemon & Coconut Chicken Curry	97
Duck Confit	97
Chicken & Mushroom	98
Seasoned Chicken	99
PORK & LAMB	**100**
Pulled Pork BBQ	100
Egg Roll Soup	100
Pork Roast w/ Apple Gravy	101
Pork Shoulder	101
Ultimate Pot Roast	102
Pork Sauerkraut	103
Pork Roast & Mushroom Gravy	103
Pulled Pork Tacos	104
Pork Chops Topped w/ Apple Balsamic	104
Kalua Pork w/ Bacon	105
Greek Ribs	105
Balsamic Rosemary Pork Tenderloin	106
Sausage & Kale	106
4-Ingredient Sausage & Cabbage	107
Kalua Pork & Cabbage	107
Lamb Leg	108
Lamb Shanks w/ Ginger & Figs	108

BEEF 110

    Beef & Broccoli 110

    Beef Short Ribs 110

    Braised Beef Short Ribs 111

    Braised Beef Ribs 111

    Smoked Maple Brisket 112

    Beef Back Ribs 112

    Corned Beef w/ Cabbage & Carrots 113

    3-Ingredient Pot Roast 114

    Corned Beef w/ Cabbage & Carrots 114

    Pot Roast 115

    Mongolian Beef with Carrots 116

    Mongolian Beef 116

    Beef Chili 117

    Very Simple 5-Ingredient Corned Beef 117

    Beef & Broccoli w/ Carrots 118

    Delicious Crispy Beef Tongue 118

    4-Ingredient Corned Beef w/ Cabbage & Carrots 119

    Beef & Broccoli 120

    Balsamic Roast Beef 120

    Italian Beef 121

    Beef Brisket 121

    2-Ingredient Ground Beef 122

Beef Barbacoa 122

STOCKS & SAUCES **124**

    Chicken Stock 124

    Beef & Chicken Bone Broth 124

    Fish & Vegetable Stock 125

    Beef Bone Broth 125

    Pork & Chicken Bone Broth 126

    Applesauce 126

    Rosemary Apple Sauce 127

    Roast Garlic 127

HOLIDAY **128**

    Sauerkraut Turkey & Sausage for New Year 128

    Pork & Sauerkraut 128

    Hot Chocolate Fondue 129

    Brussels Sprouts for the Holiday 129

    Make-Ahead Mashed Sweet Potatoes 130

    Pork Roast & Sauerkraut w/ Hotdog & Kielbasa 130

    Sweet Potato Casserole 131

    Parsnips & Caramelized Onions 132

    Make-Ahead 10-Minute Gravy 132

    Beet Borscht 133

SLOW COOKED **134**

    Slow-Cooked Kielbasa Kapusta 134

Slow Cooked Chicken w/ Sweet Potatoes & Broccoli 134

Slow-Cooked Tender Pot Roast & Holy Grail Gravy 135

Slow Cooked Roast Pork w/ Apple-Onion Gravy 135

Slow-Cooked Nomato Chili 136

Slow-Cooked Beef Short Ribs & Mushrooms 136

Slow-Cooked Rosemary-Lemon Lamb 137

SNACKS & DESSERTS...**138**

Italian Turkey-Stuffed Sweet Potatoes 138

Swedish Meatballs & Mushrooms Gravy 138

Bacon Cheesy Asparagus 139

Spinach & Garlic Beef Meatballs 139

Potato Skins w/ Bacon & Guacamole 140

Baked Apples 141

Wine "Braised" Figs on Yogurt Crème 141

Chorizo Custard 142

Vanilla Bean Cheesecake 142

Turkey Meatballs 143

Broccoli-Cauliflower Sausage Tots 144

Final Words **148**

Introduction

What Exactly Are Lectins & How to Improve Your Relationship with Gluten

LECTINS

Lectins, like gluten, are vital proteins. Plants produce lectins which act as a defense mechanism for the plant. Plants use lectins to defend them against fungi, insects and mold. Due to their agglutination ability, lectins are generally termed "agglutinins". Because lectins are resistant to digestion a lot of people believe that they are most likely dangerous in our bloodstream.

With the craving for a gluten-free diet now top priority for many, it's noteworthy to know if lectins should all together be abstained from. A common feature of lectins is their ability to remain undigested when taken, but they shouldn't be all that a no-no as some studies have shown the non-digestible "anti-nutrients" are good constituents to include in a healthy diet.

In reality, there are so many anti-nutrients from plants that abstaining from all of them altogether might leave us with little varieties to choose from when grocery shopping. Besides, they may not as inimical to our health as feared.

WHERE ARE LECTINS FOUND?

Although they are more predominant in plants, lectins can be found in animals too. Common plant sources of gluten include fruits and vegetables like eggplant, tomatoes, potatoes and peppers, as well as, egg, legumes and dairy products. Lectins are also abundant in legumes, cereal grains, almonds, soybeans and nuts, where they are chiefly present in the seeds and skins.

There probably won't be a vegan diet without lectins as they are found in just about all edible plants. And with the preposterous number of individuals suffering from diabetes and obesity – both of which are linked to more consumption of high sugar and fat diet with little or no fibers, it may be at best, an over the top measure, to rule out lectins from your diet.

Research on Lectins.

As individuals become more sensitive to foods they consume while looking for healthier alternatives, results of lectin research on the benefits or otherwise of these proteins couldn't be more interesting to find out. Many people consider lectin-free diet a perfect way to level up your energy, weight loss and acne treatment, so it's not surprising that most works have centered on finding out the impact of lectins on digestive health, inflammation and immunity among other benefits.

Gut Health

A lectin found in wheat called "wheat germ agglutinin" has been claimed to be unhealthy as it binds on the epithelial gut wall, leading to untold health problems like leaky gut syndrome due to damages on the intestinal lining. It's also believed that excessive consumption of a lectin-rich diet may predispose you to developing low nutrient absorption due to increased gut permeability as well as make pathogen defense a difficult task. Increased cell binding may also be the recipe for spontaneous episodes of pro-inflammatory immune responses and other autoimmune problems.

Intestinal diseases are likely if lectins are taken in large quantities, and more so by individuals with considerate dysfunctional enzymes. According to medics, uncooked starch present in grains and legumes provides sufficient lectins that can go on to seamlessly reach our intestinal cells, increasing the chances of coming down with food poisoning. However, as most research on lectins and their gut impact have been done on animals, a dearth of human evidence makes it slightly controversial to conclude on their effects.

The Ultimate Guide to Lectin-Free Life

Lectins have served as an impregnable defense system in plants for years. As gluten – a popular lectin takes center stage due to its presence in many foods, it's understandable why eyebrows have been raised as to the safety of lectins. But the problem is not limited to plants, with meats being another source of this controversial protein.

Generally, lectins found in nightshades, beans and legumes and in a host of other seeds and dairy products or animals are to be avoided. There are a bunch of alternatives to consider and we'll be dealing with those in the next couple of pages.

Danger Foods to Avoid

To stay healthy and safe from consuming potentially harmful components, the following foods are some you might want to consider crossing out on your next grocery checklist; Dairy, Corn, Farm animal proteins, sugars, pseudo-grains, soy, canola and other related categories of foods that may predispose you to excessive consumption of lectins.

Top 10 Tips to Stick to The Diet with Ease & Mistakes to Avoid

Sticking to a diet routine can be overly difficult without the right mindset and desire to stay away from unhealthy foods. Here are effective ways to stay on track when making a diet change.

1. **Develop good habits**

   It's not easy to make a change and stick to it, and more so when it has to do with your diet. It takes a stern resolve not to munch your delightful cake when the opportunity presents but bearing in mind the fact that sweet foods are not always sweet on your health, cutting back on harmful foods may not take longwinded months to cultivate.

2. **Motivation is key**

   In one way or the other, we all need a good reason to stay put when embarking on an arduous task. So, when it comes to your health and losing weight, it's important to write down the reasons you are making a diet change, the benefits you stand to gain therefrom and everything else you need to stay on course whenever you feel vulnerable.

3. **Eat while sitting down**

Before you take the next bite of any food, make sure to find a comfortable place to seat and be self-conscious. This way, you rule out the chances of slipping to foods you've unchecked from your plan while staying committed to only those that are beneficial for your health goals.

4. **Be your own guard**

    If you feel you won't do a tidy job alone and need some help to stick to your diet plan, make sure you report your progress on foods consumed daily to another person who shares your health goals. By consistently sending emails, voice and text messages, you surely won't want to spend time informing you made wrong choices, consequently helping you stay on course when avoiding a haphazard eating plan.

5. **Don't go with favorites**

    While it's all too common to love a particular food over others, sticking to a set diet plan will likely mean you have to contend with foods you don't particularly like. But that's the goal. To do what may not be obviously pleasing to your taste buds but invaluable for your health. Commit to only healthy foods and you should be used to your diet change in good time.

6. **Skipping foods is not as scary**

    This is not to mean you have to go for extended periods without eating. But a miss here and there may not be a bad idea for your health, too. Skip unhealthful snacks and lunch for a few days and see how well you manage the change. Hunger is not as dreaded an emergency as it may seem. If you are able to resist the urge to binge on anything when hungry, chances are that you'll go with healthful options when you decide to eat, too.

7. **Follow a strict eating regimen**

    Desserts and appetizers may be awesome but binging on milkshakes and everything that comes your way after a meal is not what you want when following a diet plan. If snacks are a must, make sure your consumption is not at the detriment of your diet. Eat when you have to eat but based on your diet plan and don't let hunger fangs dictate your regimen.

8. **Stay committed always**

    Occasionally diverting from your eating plan may not be a sin, but they add up. Real fast. And could be all that's needed to make your diet efforts fruitless. You are not only cutting on the calories but also developing a strong habit. Keep your resilience in full swing and your "give in" muscles will have a hard time sliding into unhealthful cravings.

Your 14 Day Action Plan

Day 1 – Day 9

Living a lectin-free life is surely a herculean task but following an action plan can go a long way. To begin your total boycott from lectin foods. Your first task is to go 9 days without taking the lectin-laden foods listed previously and many others with hidden toxins. Simply check the labels of your items and you'll be sure to find out if you are all clear to consume them or there are toxins to worry about. If any ingredient seems strange, look up on a trusty safe ingredients list and you should be fine. As you take this challenge in the first 9 days, you'll also want to notice your body changes and whether benefits are really adding up. Do you feel symptoms of joint and muscle pains are subsiding? How about headaches? Gut health and overall mental alertness? If you find one or more of these conditions are improving, chances are that you've avoided the harmful foods causing the distress.

Day 10

On the 10th day, we'll get back to the lectin family and start eating foods we previously avoided. Notice if your milkshakes and dairy products are reverting fuzzy feelings.

Day 11 – 12

On the 11th and 12th day, avoid the foods you took on the 10th day and notice if any changes occur. Do you experience frequent bowel movements, feel cranky than usual or have any form of worries? If you tick this checklist, then chances are your day 10 foods are the culprit and should be crossed from your diet.

Day 13

Symptoms that may have popped up after the test on day 10 should wane by the 13th day. And it's time for another test. Fancy beans, nuts and legumes? You can have them on day 13 and try out kidney beans, peanut butter and soy products, if so desired.

Day 14

You just completed your 14-day Action plan. This is the right time to evaluate your body reaction to your action plan while avoiding lectin options. If you subsequently develop strange flare-ups, you are likely to have zeroed in on the cause of your strange conditions by now. Simply ditch the lectin foods for other alternatives and you should be fine. However, if no changes occur and you feel perfectly fine, you probably don't have to cross your favorite nuts, legumes and beans from your grocery list just yet.

BREAKFAST

Boiled Eggs 3-Ways

Servings | **12**   Prep. Time | **5 minutes**   Cook Time | **3-9 minutes**
Nutritional Content (per serving): Cal | **63**   Fat | **4.4g**   Protein | **5.5g**   Carbs | **0.3g**

12 eggs (large)   1 cup water

1. Put the IP steamer basket and pour 1 cup water in the inner pot. Put the eggs in the basket. Lock the lid and close the pressure valve. Set to LOW pressure for 8-9 minutes for hard-boiled, 5-7 minutes for medium-boiled, or 3-4 minutes for soft-boiled eggs.
2. Prepare an ice bath. When the timer beeps, QPR and open the lid. With a slotted spoon, immediately transfer the eggs to the ice bath; let cool for 5 up to 10 minutes. Serve.

Egg Curry

Servings | **4**   Prep. Time | **5 minutes**   Cook Time | **25 minutes**
Nutritional Content (per serving): Cal | **268**   Fat | **20g**   Protein | **10g**   Carbs | **13g**

1 1/2 cup onion, chopped/diced
1 tablespoon lemon juice
1 teaspoon cumin seeds
1/2 cup coconut milk
1/2 tablespoon garlic, minced
1/2 tablespoon ginger, minced
1/4 cup cilantro, chopped, to garnish
2 tablespoons ghee or preferred oil
2/3 cup water, divided
6 eggs

Spices:
1 teaspoon salt, or to taste
1/2 teaspoon garam masala
1/2 teaspoon turmeric (ground)
2 teaspoons coriander powder

Whole spices (optional):
1 stick cinnamon
1 teaspoon black peppercorns
2 bay leaf
2 green cardamom

1. Set the IP to SAUTÉ MORE mode. When hot, add the oil, optional whole spices if using, and the cumin seeds. Once the cumin seeds change color, add the garlic, ginger, and onion; sauté for 3 minutes. Add the spices. Stir for 2 minutes. Add 1/3 cup of water; scrape the browned bits off the pot.
2. Carefully set the IP trivet in the pot. Put the eggs in a steel bowl; place it on the trivet. Lock the lid and close the pressure valve. Set to MANUAL HIGH pressure for 6 minutes. When the timer beeps, QPR and open the lid.
3. Carefully remove the bowl with the eggs. Put the eggs in an ice bath; peel when cool enough to handle. Pierce holes in the surface using a fork.
4. Add the remaining 1/3 cup of water and the coconut milk in the pot. Add the peeled eggs. Set the IP to SAUTÉ; simmer for 3 minutes while stirring often. Turn off the IP. Add the lemon juice. Serve garnished with the cilantro. Serve with cauliflower rice.

Tangy Greek-Style Coconut Yogurt

Servings|3   Prep. Time|**1 hour**   Cook Time|**8 hours plus 4-6 hours chilling**
Nutritional Content (per serving): Cal|**612**   Fat|**61.6g**   Protein|**10g**   Carbs|**14.5g**

1 package (5 grams) yogurt starter (dairy-free) w/ live cultures
2 cans (13.66 ounces each) coconut cream
2 tablespoons gelatin (grass-fed)
Favorite yogurt toppings, optional

Equipment:
3 pieces 1/2-pint jars w/ lids

1. Pour the coconut cream into your IP inner pot. Press YOGUR and press ADJUST to boil the coconut cream. When the LED display shows YOGURT, remove the inner pot from the housing; turn off your IP. Let the coconut cream cool to just below 100F – the live cultures will, not grow if the temperature is not correct. Gradually add the yogurt starter to mix without making any lumps.
2. Return the inner pot to the housing, set to YOGURT for 8 hours. The longer the cooking time, the tangier it will become. When the timer beeps, QPR and open the lid. While the yogurt is still warm, gradually whisk in the gelatin to mix without making any lumps.
3. Divide the yogurt between the pint jars; leave enough room for toppings. Alternatively, you can put the toppings in the jars first before adding the yogurt. Screw the lids on; refrigerate for 4 up to 6 hours.

Cheese & Bacon Muffins

Servings|4   Prep. Time|**15 minutes**   Cook Time|**8 minutes**
Nutritional Content (per serving): Cal|**127**   Fat|**9.4g**   Protein|**9.7g**   Carbs|**0.9g**

1 1/2 cup water, for the IP
1 green onion, diced
1/4 teaspoon lemon pepper seasoning
4 eggs
4 slices bacon (grass-fed), cooked & crumbled

4 tablespoons real parmesan (parmegiano reggiano) cheese, shredded

Equipment:
4 silicone muffin cups

1. Put the IP trivet and pour the water into the inner pot. Break the eggs into a measuring bowl, preferably large with a pout. Add the seasoning; beat well. Divide the bacon, parmesan, and green onion between the muffin cups. Pour the egg mixture into the cups. Place the cups on the trivet. Lock the lid and close the pressure valve. Set to HIGH pressure for 8 minutes.
2. When the timer beeps, press CANCEL, NPR for 2 minutes, then QPR and open the lid. Remove the muffins from the IP. Serve. Refrigerate leftovers for 1 week. Microwave on HIGH for 30 seconds to reheat.

Crustless Spinach Quiche

Servings|6   Prep. Time|**15 minutes**   Cook Time|**20 minutes**
Nutritional Content (per serving): Cal|**179**   Fat|**11.2g**   Protein|**15.3g**   Carbs|**5g**

1 1/2 cup water, for the IP
1 cup preferred lectin-free veggies (cauliflower, broccoli, mushrooms, diced, with extra to top the quiche
1/2 cup coconut milk
1/2 teaspoon salt
1/4 cup real parmesan (parmegiano reggiano) cheese, shredded
1/4 teaspoon black pepper (fresh ground)

12 eggs (large)
3 cups baby spinach (fresh), roughly chopped
3 green onions (large), sliced

Equipment:
1 1/2-quart baking dish

1. Put the IP trivet and pour the water into the inner pot. In a bowl, preferably large, whisk the eggs, milk, salt, and pepper. Add the spinach, preferred veggies, and green onions in the baking dish; stir to mix well.
2. Put the dish on the trivet. Lock the lid and close the pressure valve. Set to HIGH pressure for 20 minutes. When the timer beeps, press CANCEL, NPR for 10 minutes, QPR, and open the lid. Remove the dish from the pot. If preferred, broil the quiche till the top is light brown.
NOTES: You can cook the quiche uncovered. Just soak the moisture on the top with paper towels. Or, you can cover the dish with foil to prevent the moisture from gathering on the quiche.

Sweet Potato Hash w/ Mushrooms

Servings|2   Prep. Time|**20 minutes**   Cook Time|**5-6 minutes**
Nutritional Content (per serving): Cal|**393**   Fat|**7.9g**   Protein|**6.5g**   Carbs|**55.6g**

1 clove garlic, minced
1 tablespoon olive oil
1 teaspoon cumin
1 teaspoon paprika
1/2 cup mushrooms, chopped
1/2 cup water

1/2 teaspoon black pepper (fresh ground)
1/2 teaspoon salt (kosher)
2 sweet potato (large), cut into 1-inch chunks (around 2 cups)

1. Toss your veggies with the oil and then the spices. Put them in the inner pot. Add the water. Lock the lid and close the pressure valve. Set to HIGH pressure for 25 minutes. When the timer beeps, QPR and open the lid.
2. Press SAUTÉ; fry the veggies for 5 up to 6 minutes or till the potato cubes start to brown. Serve. If preferred, top with sunny-side-up eggs.

Eggs En Cocotte

Servings|3   Prep. Time|**10 minutes**   Cook Time|**2-4 minutes**
Nutritional Content (per serving): Cal|**173**   Fat|**16.6g**   Protein|**5.8g**   Carbs|**0.8g**

1 cup water, for the IP
1 tablespoon chives
3 eggs (fresh, pasture raised)
3 tablespoons heavy cream, divided
Butter, at room temperature

Sea salt & pepper (freshly ground)

Equipment:
3 pieces 4 or 5-ounce ramekins

1. Grease the sides and bottoms of the ramekins with butter. Pour 1 tablespoon of cream into each. Carefully crack an egg over the cream, making sure to keep the yolks intact; sprinkle with the chives.

2. Put the IP trivet and pour the water into the inner pot. Put the ramekins on the rack. Lock the lid and close the pressure valve. Set to MANUAL LOW pressure for 4 minutes for firm yolks or for 2 minutes for runny yolks. When the timer beeps, QPR and open the lid. Season the eggs en cocotte with pepper and salt. Serve.
NOTES: If cooking less than 3 servings, fill the remaining ramekins with water and put them in the pot as well. Otherwise, the eggs will cook too fast.

Tapioca Pearl Pudding

Servings|**4-6**   Prep. Time|**5 minutes**   Cook Time|**20 minutes**
Nutritional Content (per serving): Cal|**186**   Fat|**2.5g**   Protein|**2.5g**   Carbs|**40.7g**

1 1/4 cups coconut milk (300 grams)
1 cup water, for the IP
1/2 cup stevia (100 grams)
1/2 cup water (115 grams)
1/2 lemon, zested

1/3 cup pearl sago/tapioca pearls (60 grams)

Equipment:
4-cup heatproof bowl

1. Put the IP trivet and pour the water into the inner pot. Put the rest of the ingredients in the bowl; mix till the stevia is fully dissolved. Put the bowl on the trivet. Lock the lid and close the pressure valve. Set to HIGH pressure for 8 minutes.

2. When the timer beeps, press CANCEL, NPR completely, around 20 up to 30 minutes, then QPR and open the lid. Carefully remove the bowl from the pot. With a fork, vigorously stir the contents. Divide between 4-6 bowls or glasses. Serve as is or top with preferred seasonal fruits.

Bacon & Sausage Omelet

Servings|6   Prep. Time|**20 minutes**   Cook Time|**25 minutes**
Nutritional Content (per serving): Cal|**222**   Fat|**15.5g**   Protein|**16.8g**   Carbs|**3.5g**

1 onion, diced
1/2 cup coconut milk
6 fresh sausages links, sliced
6 slices bacon, cooked
6 up to 12 eggs
Cooking spray (olive oil)
Garlic powder
Pepper

Salt
16 ounces water, for the IP
Parmesan cheese, shredded
Oregano (dried)

Equipment:
1 1/2-quart Pyrex or ceramic baking dish
Measuring cup (large)

1. Crack the eggs in a measuring cup. Add the milk; whisk using a hand mixer till well combined. Add the onion and sausages; season to taste with pepper, salt, and garlic powder. Grease the baking dish/Pyrex with the cooking spray. Pour the egg mixture into the dish; tightly cover with foil.

2. Put the IP trivet and pour the water into the inner pot. Put the baking dish on the trivet. Lock the lid and close the pressure valve. Set to MANUAL HIGH pressure for 25 minutes. When the timer beeps, press CANCEL, NPR completely, then QPR and open the lid.

3. Remove the foil. If the egg popped out of the dish, then just push it back. Layer the cooked bacon on top of the egg mixture. Cover with the parmesan cheese. Lock the lid and close the pressure valve. Set to MANUAL HIGH pressure for 5 minutes. Remove the dish from the pot. Sprinkle with some oregano (dried). Slice into portions; serve.

Crustless Meaty Quiche

Servings|4   Prep. Time|**15 minutes**   Cook Time|**30 minutes**
Nutritional Content (per serving): Cal|**419**   Fat|**31.3g**   Protein|**29.6g**   Carbs|**4.1g**

1 1/2 cups water, for the IP
1 cup cheese, shredded
1 cup ground sausage, cooked
1/2 cup ham, diced
1/2 cup milk
1/4 teaspoon salt
1/8 teaspoon black pepper (fresh ground)

2 green onions (large), chopped
4 slices bacon, cooked & crumbled
6 eggs (large), well beaten

Equipment:
1-quart soufflé dish

1. Put the IP trivet and pour the water into the inner pot. In a bowl, preferably large, whisk the eggs, milk, pepper, and salt. Put the ham, bacon, sausage, and green onion in the soufflé dish;

mix well. Pour the egg mixture over the meat mixture; stir to mix well. Loosely cover the dish with foil.

2. Put the dish on the trivet. Lock the lid and close the pressure valve. Set to HIGH pressure for 30 minutes. When the timer beeps, press CANCEL, NPR for 10 minutes, then QPR and open the lid. Remove the dish from the pot; remove the foil. If preferred, sprinkle the top of the quiche with extra cheese; broil till the cheese is melted and slightly brown. Serve.

Egg Custard

Servings|4-5   Prep. Time|4 minutes   Cook Time|6 minutes
Nutritional Content (per serving): Cal|119   Fat|4g   Protein|5g   Carbs|13g

1 1/2 cup (375 ml) coconut milk, divided
3 eggs (large), around 180 ml volume
4-5 tablespoons stevia
Pinch salt

1 cup cold water, for the IP

Equipment:
4 or 5 pieces (3x1 1/2-inch) ramekins

1. Using the SLOW COOK mode of the IP, melt the sugar and pinch of salt with 1 cup of the milk; stirring with a silicone spatula till fully dissolved. Remove the inner pot from the housing. Add the remaining milk; mix well – it should be cool to touch at this point.

2. In a measuring cup, preferably large, whisk the eggs till well mixed. While continuously whisking, gradually add the milk mixture to the eggs; mix well. Strain the beaten eggs 2 times through a strainer (fine mesh) to remove any solids and make it smooth. Divide the egg mixture between the ramekins; remove any bubble using a spoon. Cover the ramekins with foil very tightly.

3. Wash the inner pot, dry well, and return to the housing. Put the IP trivet and pour the water into the inner pot. Put the ramekins on the trivet, stacking them in 2 layers if needed. Lock the lid and close the pressure valve. Set to LOW pressure for 0 minutes at sea level or 1 minute if above sea level or if the foil you are using is thick. When the timer beeps, press CANCEL, NPR for 10 minutes, then QPR and open the lid. Remove the ramekins from the oven and set aside to avoid overcooking. Serve while still hot or warm.

Ham Casserole

Servings|4-6   Prep. Time|20 minutes   Cook Time|25 minutes
Nutritional Content (per serving): Cal|621   Fat|38.7g   Protein|30.8g   Carbs|39g

1 cup coconut milk
1 cup ham, chopped
1 teaspoon pepper
1 teaspoon salt

1/2 onion, diced
10 eggs (large)
2 cups parmesan cheese, shredded

4 sweet potatoes (medium), peeled & chunked

2 cups water, for the IP

1. Grease a heatproof container that will fit your IP with lectin-free cooking spray. Put the milk and eggs in the bowl; whisk till well mixed. Add the potatoes, cheese, ham, onion, pepper, and salt; stir to mix well and everything is covered with the egg mixture. Cover the container with foil.

2. Put the IP trivet and pour the water into the inner pot. Put the container in the trivet. Lock the lid and close the pressure valve. Set to MANUAL for 25 minutes. When the timer beeps, QPR and open the lid. Serve with preferred lectin-free toppings, such as sour cream and avocado. Season with pepper and salt as needed.

Twice-Baked Sweet Potatoes Casserole

Servings|6-10   Prep. Time|20-25 minutes   Cook Time|40-45 minutes
Nutritional Content (per serving): Cal|852   Fat|52g   Protein|22g   Carbs|78g

1 1/2 sticks butter
1 bundle green onions chopped
1 cup coconut milk (may need more to make it creamier)
1 cup sour cream
1 ranch seasoning mix

2 cups parmesan cheese, shredded, with extra for topping
4 slices bacon, cooked & crumbled
5 pounds sweet potatoes
Pepper & salt to taste
1 cup water

1. Slice the potatoes into chunks; leave the skins on. Put them in your IP. Add the water, 1 stick of butter, pepper, and salt. Lock the lid and close the pressure valve. Set to MANUAL for 6 minutes. When the timer beeps, QPR and open the lid.
2. Add the milk and butter. Mash the mixture using a hand masher or an electric hand mixer right in the pot. Add the ranch seasoning and sour cream; mix well. Fold in the parmesan and green onions.
3. Transfer the potato mixture to a baking dish. Top with extra cheese, bacon, and chives. Bake for 20 minutes at 350F.

Frosted Egg Frittata Cupcakes

Servings|4   Prep. Time|5 minutes   Cook Time|5 minutes
Nutritional Content (per serving): Cal|229   Fat|18.4g   Protein|11g   Carbs|5.3g

1 cup water, for the IP
1 scallion, diced, reserve half
1 tablespoon heavy cream
1/2 cup cheese, diced/shredded

1/2 cup sweet potatoes, peeled & finely diced
1/2 teaspoon preferred seasoning mix

1/4 cup bacon, diced & crisped
7 eggs (large)

Equipment:
4 pieces half-pint mason jars, well-greased

1. Mix the eggs, cream, and seasoning; divide the mixture between the mason jars. Mix the 1/4 cup of cheese, 1/2 of the scallions, bacon, and potatoes; divide between the mason jars.

2. Put the IP trivet and pour the water into the inner pot. Put the mason jars on the trivet. Lock the lid and close the pressure valve. Set to HIGH pressure for 5 minutes. When the timer beeps, press CANCEL, NPR for 10 minutes, then QPR and open the lid.
Frost the top of each frittata with grated cheese. Close the lid; let sit for 1 minute. Remove the mason jars from the pot; garnish with the scallions.

Oef en Cocotte a.k.a French "Baked" Eggs

Servings|4   Prep. Time|5 minutes   Cook Time|8 minutes
Nutritional Content (per serving): Cal|**175**   Fat|**21g**   Protein|**14g**   Carbs|**2g**

4 eggs
4 garnishes fresh herbs
4 slices parmesan cheese or shots of heavy cream
4 slices preferred lectin-free fish, meat, or veggies

Olive oil
1 cup water, for the IP

Equipment:
4 pieces 3 or 4-ounce ramekins

1. Put the IP trivet and pour the water into the inner pot. Grease the sides and bottoms of the ramekins with the olive oil. Lay 1 slice of preferred lectin-free fish, meat, or veggies in each ramekin; break 1 egg into each. Top with cheese of heavy cream. Leave the ramekins uncovered for hard-cooked yolks or cover with foil tightly for soft yolks.

2. Put the ramekins on the trivet. Lock the lid and close the pressure valve. Set to LOW pressure for 4 minutes. When the timer beeps, QPR and open the lid. Transfer the ramekins to individual saucers or little plates. Serve.

Scotch Eggs

Servings|4   Prep. Time|15 minutes   Cook Time|12 minutes
Nutritional Content (per serving): Cal|**252**   Fat|**43.44g**   Protein|**18.86g**   Carbs|**1.35g**

1 pound ground sausage (country-style)
1 tablespoon oil

4 eggs (large)
2 cups water, for the IP

1. Put the IP steamer basket and pour 1 cup water in the inner pot. Put the eggs in the basket. Lock the lid and close the pressure valve. Set to HIGH pressure for 6 minutes.

2. When the timer beeps, press CANCEL, NPR for 6 minutes, then QPR and open the lid. Remove the steamer basket from the pot. Transfer the eggs to an ice bath and cool. When they are cool, peel the shells.

3. Divide the sausage into 4 equal portions; flatten each into a flat round. Put an egg in the center and then wrap the sausage around the egg gently. Set the IP to SAUTÉ. When hot, add the oil. Add the Scotch eggs and cook till all the sides are brown. Remove the eggs from the pot. Add 1 cup of water. Put the IP steamer basket in the inner pot. Place the eggs on the basket.

4. Lock the lid and close the pressure valve. Set to HIGH pressure for 6 minutes. When the timer beeps, QPR and open the lid. Serve your Scotch eggs.

Slow Cooked Ham & Spinach Frittata

Servings|8   Prep. Time|15-20 minutes   Cook Time|2-3 or 4-6 hours
Nutritional Content (per serving): Cal|191   Fat|14g   Protein|13g   Carbs|4g

1 cup ham, diced
1 onion (small), chopped
1 teaspoon coconut oil
1 teaspoon sea salt
1/2 cup coconut milk (canned)
1/2 teaspoon pepper
2 cloves garlic
2 cups spinach, chopped
8 eggs, beaten

1. Set the IP to SAUTÉ normal mode. Add the oil. When hot, add the onion and garlic; cook till soft. Press CANCEL. Add the ham and spinach; stir to mix.
2. In a bowl, preferably medium, whisk the eggs, milk, pepper, and salt till mixed well. Add to the IP. Lock the lid and close the pressure valve. Set to SLOW COOK for 4 up to 6 hours on LOW or for 2 up to 3 hours on HIGH or till the eggs are set. Serve hot.

Sweet Potato Hash

Servings|4   Prep. Time|10 minutes   Cook Time|10 minutes
Nutritional Content (per serving): Cal|312   Fat|18g   Protein|24g   Carbs|13.4g

1 onion (small), peeled & diced
1 sweet potato (large), peeled & cubed
1 tablespoon Italian seasoning
1/2 pound pork sausage (ground)
1/2 teaspoon black pepper (fresh ground)
1/2 teaspoon sea salt

2 cloves garlic, minced
2 cups water, for the IP
6 eggs (large)

Equipment:
7-cup glass dish, greased well

1. In a bowl, preferably medium, whisk the eggs, pepper, salt, and Italian seasoning; set aside. Set the IP to SAUTÉ. Stir-fry the onion, garlic, sweet potato, and sausage for 3 minutes or till the onions are translucent. Transfer the mixture to the glass dish. Pour the egg mixture over the meat mixture.

2. Put the IP trivet and pour the water into the inner pot. Put the dish on the trivet. Lock the lid and close the pressure valve. Set to MANUAL HIGH pressure for 5 minutes. When the timer beeps, QPR and open the lid. Transfer the dish to a heatproof surface; let sit for 5 minutes at room temperature to allow the eggs to set. Slice into portions; serve.

Sausage Egg Casserole

Servings|12   Prep. Time|**5 minutes**   Cook Time|**5 minutes**
Nutritional Content (per serving): Cal|**315**   Fat|**23g**   Protein|**20g**   Carbs|**5g**

1 3/4 cups ground sausage, cooked
1/2 teaspoons black pepper (fresh ground)
1/2 teaspoons garlic salt
12 eggs

2 cups parmesan cheese, shredded
1 cup water, for the IP

Equipment:
12 silicone muffins cups, well-greased

1. Put the IP trivet and pour the water into the inner pot. Mix all of the ingredients in a bowl, preferably large. Pour the mixture into the muffin cups. Put the cups on the trivet. Lock the lid and close the pressure valve. Set to HIGH pressure for 5 minutes. When the timer beeps, QPR and open the lid. Serve.

Slow Cooked Breakfast Chicken Soup

Servings|0   Prep. Time|**10 minutes**   Cook Time|**10 hours**
Nutritional Content (per serving): Cal|**683**   Fat|**45g**   Protein|**44g**   Carbs|**24g**

1 whole chicken
2 1/2 quarts water, chicken stock, or bone broth
Salt (fine sea), to taste

For each serving of soup:
1/2 avocado, chopped
2 tablespoons Italian parsley or cilantro (fresh), chopped
2 tablespoons scallions, chopped

1. Put the chicken in your IP. Add the cooking liquid over it. Lock the lid and close the pressure valve. Set to SLOW COOK for 10 hours or till the meat is fall-off-the-bone.

2. When the chicken is cooked, transfer to a large plate. Pull the meat from the bone using a fork and return to the pot; save the bones to make bone broth. Season the soup as needed with salt. Add avocado, parsley/cilantro, and fresh herbs to each serving.

Sweet Potato & Collard Hash

Servings|4   Prep. Time|25 minutes   Cook Time|35-40 minutes
Nutritional Content (per serving): Cal|166   Fat|10g   Protein|30g   Carbs|4g

1 bunch collards, stemmed & roughly chopped
1 cup red onion, finely diced
1 teaspoon salt (kosher)
1/2 cup chicken stock
1/2 teaspoon black pepper (fresh ground)
1/2 teaspoon paprika (smoked sweet)
2 sweet potatoes (medium), peeled & small diced
2 tablespoons olive oil

1. Set the IP to SAUTE. Add the olive oil. When hot, add the onion and garlic; cook for 4 minutes or till almost translucent. Add the potatoes; cook for 5 minutes or till golden. Add the collards; cook for 5 minutes or till wilted. Add the pepper, salt, and paprika; cook for 1 minute.

2. Add the broth. Lock the lid and close the pressure valve. Set to MANUAL HIGH for 6 minutes. When the timer beeps, QPR and open the lid. Set the IP to SAUTE. Cook for 3 minutes to reduce the cooking liquid and re-crisp the outside of the potatoes.

Breakfast Casserole

Servings|6   Prep. Time|0 minutes   Cook Time|0 minutes
Nutritional Content (per serving): Cal|228   Fat|17.5g   Protein|12.5g   Carbs|5g

8 egg
2/3 cups sweet potato, peeled & grated
2 teaspoons garlic cloves, minced
2 tablespoons coconut oil
1 cup kale, chopped
1 1/3 cups leek, sliced
1 1/2 cups water
1 1/2 cups sausage breakfast, cooked

1. Set the IP to SAUTE. Add the coconut oil. When melted, add the garlic, leeks, and kale; saute till soft. Remove the sautéed veggies from the inner pot and clean.

2. In a bowl (large), mix the eggs, sautéed veggies, sausage, and sweet potato. Pour the mixture into greased ovenproof bowl/pan. Put the IP trivet and pour the water into the inner pot. Put

the bowl/pan on the trivet. Lock the lid and close the pressure valve. Set to HIGH pressure for 25 minutes. When the timer beeps, QPR and open the lid. Remove the bowl/pan from the pot. Slice into equal portions; serve.

Is your belly happy yet?

We sincerely hope that you're pleased with the recipes so far. If not, feel free to send us an email at info@limitlessrecipes.com and tell us what we can improve. We get back to every person who reaches out.

If you are enjoying the recipes then you will love the box set below with over 600 delicious and easy to make recipes.

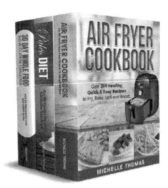

Only sign up for the cookbook box set if you are ready to be absolutely amazed with over 600 proven, delicious and easy to make recipes.

To access the gift page type in www.bit.ly/2Ho82AH or email us at info@limitlessrecipes.com to get the box set delivered to your email.

Limitless Recipes
Like us on Facebook and join our private Facebook group community for more recipes and gifts.
@limitlessrecipes
Follow us on Instagram
Limitless Recipes
Follow us on Pinterest.

Want to be a part of our closed Facebook group?
We are working on building an engaged community discussing recipes and healthy eating in our closed Facebook group. If you would like to be involved in the discussions about cooking, what is working, what is not working and receive information about gifts and promotions, we would be delighted to add you.

Type in Limitless Recipes on Facebook or write us at info@limitlessrecipes.com. Come say hi!

Happy Cooking!

Can we ask you for a quick favor?

We try to write the best cookbooks that we can and a lot of effort goes into writing the cookbook with so many recipes while making sure that the recipes are healthy and fairly easy to make. We sincerely hope you are enjoying the recipes. That being said, reviews really help us A LOT when it comes to putting our names out there and keep us motivated. Competing with big publishing companies is quite hard and reviews really help with making our books more visible.
If you could take one minute to leave a review, we would really appreciate that.

You can leave a review in 3 easy steps:
1. Go to the product page
2. Scroll down and on the left side click 'Write customer review'
3. Write a review and click 'Submit'

Thank you so much. **You are amazing!**

If you feel like we could improve the cookbook please email us at info@limitlessrecipes.com and we'll make sure to get back to you.

Feel free to proceed to the lunch recipes, yummy!

LUNCH

Southwest Chicken w/ Cauliflower Rice

Servings|**4**   Prep. Time|**20 minutes**   Cook Time|**30 minutes**
Nutritional Content (per serving): Cal|**651**   Fat|**21.4g**   Protein|**101.4g**   Carbs|**10.2g**

1 head cauliflower, broken into large chunks
1 tablespoon butter/ghee
2 tablespoons coconut oil
2-3 pounds chicken hindquarters, thighs, or legs (bone-in)
Pepper (fresh ground)

For the spice rub:
1 tablespoon garlic powder
1 tablespoon sea salt (Himalayan pink)
1 teaspoon black pepper (fresh ground)
2 teaspoons coriander
2 teaspoons cumin
2 teaspoons onion powder
2 teaspoons oregano
2 teaspoons paprika (smoked)

1. Chicken: Pat dry the chicken using paper towels. In a bowl, mix all of the spice rub ingredients. Rub all the sides of the chicken with the spice mixture; reserve a small amount for your cauliflower.

2. Add butter/ghee in the IP. Set it to SAUTÉ. Add the chicken; cook till brown. Transfer the browned chicken to a bowl. Add 1/2 cup of water in the pot; scrape the browned bits from the pot using a wooden spoon. Carefully put the trivet in the IP. Put the chicken on the trivet.

3. Lock the lid and close the pressure valve. Set to MANUAL HIGH pressure for 12 or 13 minutes for thighs or for 10 minutes for drumsticks. When the timer beeps, QPR and open the lid. Turn off the IP.

4. Carefully transfer the chicken to a serving dish. Cover the dish with foil to keep warm. Wearing an oven mitt, remove the trivet from the IP. Scoop out the cooking liquid from the pot, leaving 1 cup. Return the trivet.

5. Cauliflower: Put the cauliflower on the trivet. Lock the lid and close the pressure valve. Set to HIGH pressure for 1 minute. When the timer beeps, QPR and open the lid. Carefully remove the trivet with cauliflower from the pot. Turn off the IP. Wearing an oven mitt, carefully lift the inner pot from the housing; pour the cooking liquid out, and then return it to the housing.

6. Set the IP to SAUTÉ. Add the butter and cooked cauliflower. Using a potato masher, break the cauliflower chunks. Add the reserved spice mixture. Sauté till the cauliflower resembles rice. Turn off the IP. Serve with the chicken.

Alaska Cod Tacos w/ Lime-Garlic Sour Cream

Servings | 6   Prep. Time | **15 minutes**   Cook Time | **15 minutes**
Nutritional Content (per serving): Cal | **265**   Fat | **13g**   Protein | **14g**   Carbs | **23g**

Fish:
1 pound frozen (loin fillets) Alaska cod
1 tablespoon lime juice (fresh)
1 tablespoon olive oil
1 teaspoon cumin
1/2 teaspoon coriander
1/2 teaspoon paprika (smoked)
1/2 teaspoon salt (kosher)

Sour cream:
1/2 cup sour cream
2 tablespoon cilantro, chopped
1/2 teaspoon lime zest
1 teaspoon lime juice
1/4 teaspoon salt (kosher)
1 garlic clove, minced

Other:
Cabbage, chopped
Cilantro, snipped
Lime, for squeezing on tacos

1. Fish: Get a 24-inch piece of foil or parchment paper. Put the fish filler in the middle. Evenly drizzle them with the lime juice and olive oil. Sprinkle with the salt, paprika, coriander, and cumin. Bring the sides of the foil up; fold down 2 times. Double fold both ends of the foil to seal the packet; leave a space for the heat to circulate.

2. Put the IP trivet and pour 1 cup water in the inner pot. Put the packet on the trivet. Lock the lid and close the pressure valve. Set to MANUAL for 8 minutes. When the timer beeps, QPR and open the lid. The fish is done when the flesh flakes easily when tested with a fork.

3. Remove the packet from the pot. Open it. Transfer the fish and the juices to a mixing bowl; break the fish into pieces using 2 forks. Season as needed.

4. Sour cream: Mix the garlic, salt, lime juice, lime zest, cilantro, and sour cream in a bowl; refrigerate till using. Prepare your preferred toppings. Top the fish with the sour cream and cabbage; drizzle with lime juice.

Creamy Chicken Soup

Servings|0   Prep. Time|5 minutes   Cook Time|50 minutes
Nutritional Content (per serving): Cal|484   Fat|377g   Protein|22.6g   Carbs|17.1g

1 avocado, diced
8 ounce (bagged) Mann's Kale and Beet blend
1 can coconut milk (full-fat)
1 onion, diced
1 pound chicken thighs (skinless & boneless)
1 tablespoon avocado oil

1 teaspoon fish sauce
1 teaspoon garlic powder
1 teaspoon salt
1 teaspoon thyme (dried)
2 tablespoons sesame oil (optional)
2/3 cup bone broth, divided
4 cloves garlic, minced
Juice of 1 lemon

1. Set the IP to SAUTE. Add the oil, onion, and garlic; sauté for 8 minutes or till soft. Move the onion mixture to one side of the IP. Add the chicken to the cleared side; make sure it touches the bottom of the pot. Cook each side for 6 minutes or till both sides are brown. Mix it with the onion mixture.

2. Add 1/3 cup of broth and the seasoning. Lock the lid and close the pressure valve. Set to HIGH pressure for 5 minutes. When the timer beeps, QPR and open the lid.

3. Shred the chicken using 2 forks. Add the rest of the broth, lemon juice, coconut milk, and the kale and beet blend. Lock the lid and close the pressure valve. Set to HIGH pressure for 2 minutes. When the timer beeps, QPR and open the lid. Stir well and serve. Garnish with the optional sesame oil if using and diced avocado.

One-Pot Pork Belly & Spiced Cauliflower Rice

Servings|4   Prep. Time|15 minutes   Cook Time|15 minutes
Nutritional Content (per serving): Cal|639   Fat|62g   Protein|14g   Carbs|8g

1 pound pork belly, cooked & cubed
4 cups cauliflower rice
1/2 cup bone broth
1/2 red onion, sliced
1/2 cup cilantro, divided
2 green onions, sliced
1 tablespoon lime juice

3 cloves garlic, sliced
1 tablespoon bacon fat
1 teaspoon turmeric
1 tablespoon oregano
1 tablespoon cumin, optional
1/2 teaspoon salt

1. Except for 1/4 cup of cilantro, put all the ingredients in the IP. Lock the lid and close the pressure valve. Set to MANUAL for 15 minutes. When the timer beeps, press CANCEL, NPR for 10 minutes, then QPR and open the lid. Serve topped with the remaining cilantro.

Pear & Almond Chicken Lettuce Wraps

Servings|4   Prep. Time|**15 minutes**   Cook Time|**20 minutes**
Nutritional Content (per serving): Cal|**711**   Fat|**48g**   Protein|**47g**   Carbs|**26g**

Chicken:
1 cup bone or chicken broth
2 pounds chicken thighs (skinless & boneless)
Pepper & salt

Wraps:
1 tablespoon fish sauce
1 pear (Asian), cored & diced
1/4 cup almond butter
2 carrots, grated
1 tablespoon white vinegar
2 lettuce heads (romaine, Bibb, or butter)
Juice of 1 lime

1. Chicken: Put everything ingredients in your IP. Lock the lid and close the pressure valve. Set to MANUAL for twenty (20) minutes. When the timer beeps, QPR and open the lid. Transfer the chicken to a large plate or cutting board; shred using 2 forks. Discard the broth or save for other uses.
2. Lettuce wraps: Put the carrots and pear to a mixing bowl. Add the chicken, vinegar, lime juice, fish sauce, and almond butter. Mix till well combined. Put chicken mixture into lettuce leaves; wrap and serve.

Chicken Lettuce Wraps

Servings|4   Prep. Time|**8 minutes**   Cook Time|**27 minutes**
Nutritional Content (per serving): Cal|**341**   Fat|**19g**   Protein|**26g**   Carbs|**16g**

1 pound ground chicken
1/2 cups water chestnuts (canned), drained & sliced
1/2 teaspoons ginger (ground)
1/3 cups green onion (scallion), sliced
1/4 cups chicken broth/stock
1/4 cups coconut aminos
1/8 teaspoons allspice (ground)
2 tablespoons balsamic vinegar
3/4 cups onion, diced
5 teaspoons garlic cloves, minced
8 individual romaine lettuce

1. Put all the ingredients in your IP in the following order: chicken, onion, garlic, ginger, allspice, water chestnuts, coconut aminos, and broth/stock. Lock the lid and close the pressure valve. Set to HIGH pressure for 10 minutes. When the timer beeps, QPR and open the lid. With a meat masher or fork, break the chunks of meat. Spoon the meat mixture into the lettuce leaves; garnish with the green onions. Serve.

Loaded Beef Stew

Servings|6   Prep. Time|**15 minutes**   Cook Time|**50 minutes**
Nutritional Content (per serving): Cal|**428**   Fat|**11.5g**   Protein|**41g**   Carbs|**43g**

4 stalks parsley (fresh), chopped
3 tablespoons sherry vinegar or fish sauce
3 stalks celery, chopped into 1/4-inch pieces
3 sprigs thyme (fresh)
3 shallots (small) or 1 onion (medium), around 1/2 cups
3 cups mushrooms (cremini), thinly sliced
3 carrots (medium), peeled & chopped into 1/2-inch rounds
3 sweet potatoes (medium), peeled & chopped into 1/2-inch chunks
2 teaspoons salt (kosher)
2 tablespoons tapioca flour mixed w/ 1/4 cup warm water
2 tablespoons avocado oil, divided
2 pounds stewing beef
2 cups parsnips, peeled & chopped into 1/2-inch rounds
2 bay leaf (dried)
1/2 teaspoon pepper (fresh ground)
1 liter beef stock

1. Set the IP to SAUTE. Add 1 tablespoon of avocado oil. Season the beef with pepper and salt. When the oil is warm, cook the beef in 2 batches till all the sides are brown. Transfer the browned meat to a bowl; set aside.

2. Add the remaining oil to the pot. Add the carrots, mushrooms, celery, shallot, and thyme; saute for 2 minutes or till the shallot is translucent. Add 2 tablespoons wine/fish sauce to deglaze the IP; scrape the browned bits off the pot. Add the potatoes, parsnips, and beef, along with any accumulated meat juices.

3. In a bowl or glass (small), mix the flour with the warm water till smooth. Add the broth, bay leaves, and flour mixture to the pot. Season with 1 teaspoon pepper and salt. Lock the lid and close the pressure valve. Set to MANUAL HIGH pressure for 30 minutes. When the timer beeps, press CANCEL, NPR for 20 minutes, then QPR and open the lid. Remove the bay leaves. Season with pepper and salt as needed. Add 1 tablespoon wine. Top each serving with parsley.

One-Pot Roast & Sweet Potato-Cauliflower Mash

Servings|4   Prep. Time|**10 minutes**   Cook Time|**35 minutes**
Nutritional Content (per serving): Cal|**653**   Fat|**26.4g**   Protein|**70.2g**   Carbs|**31.7g**

3/4 cup water
3 tablespoons Dijon mustard
3 sweet potatoes, (medium), peeled & roughly diced
2-3 pound pork loin roast
2 tablespoons yogurt (plain)
2 sprigs thyme (fresh)
2 sprigs sage (fresh)
2 sprigs mint (fresh)
1/2 teaspoon salt
1/2 teaspoon pepper
1 tablespoon olive oil
1 cauliflower head (medium), separated into florets (large)
1 bouquet edible flowers (untreated), such as Alyssum & dandelions

1. Put the potato and cauliflower in a heatproof bowl. Tie 1 sprig of each herb to the pork; paint it with the mustard. Set the IP to SAUTÉ NORMAL mode. When hot, add the oil and roast; cook till all the sides are brown. When all the sides of the meat are browned, add the broth; season with pepper and salt. Set the bowl, with the veggies on top of the pork. If needed, balance it by placing ball/s of crumbled foil on the base to keep it somewhat upright.

2. Lock the lid and close the pressure valve. Set to MANUAL HIGH pressure for 30 minutes. When the timer beeps, press CANCEL, NPR for 10 minutes, then QPR and open the lid.

3. Remove the bowl from the pot; wipe the base and sides dry using paper towels. Add the yogurt to the bowl; mash the contents. Transfer the pork to a cutting board; slice into thin pieces and put the slices into a serving dish. Wet the pork slices with the cooking juices and then garnish with the edible flowers and remaining herbs. Serve.

Pulled-Pork Chipotle Salad

Servings|4   Prep. Time|**30 minutes**   Cook Time|**1 hour, 30 minutes**
Nutritional Content (per serving): Cal|**1459**   Fat|**111g**   Protein|**106.5g**   Carbs|**3g**

1 pinch oregano (dried) leaves
1 teaspoon black pepper (fresh ground)
1 teaspoon garlic powder
1 teaspoon paprika (smoked) powder
2 cups chicken stock
2 teaspoons sea salt
4 pounds pork shoulder or butt meat, or 7 pounds (on-the-bone) shoulder
4 tablespoons coconut oil
6 cloves garlic

1. Remove the rinds from your pork; slice the meat from the bone if using on-the-bone shoulder. Slice the meat into large chunks. Trim any fat off. Set the IP to SAUTÉ. Add the oil. When hot, add just enough pork meat to cover the bottom of your pot; cook till some spots are nicely browned.

2. While the meat is browning, peel your garlic and slice them into small chunks. Transfer the browned meat to a bowl (large). Add a couple tablespoons stock in the IP; scrape the browned bits off the pot using a wooden spoon. Transfer the broth and scraped browned bits mixture to the bowl with the browned meat. Continue cooking the rest of the meat following the same process, setting the IP to SAUTÉ again as needed to brown all the meat.

3. When all the meat is browned and in the bowl, add the salt, pepper, garlic powder, paprika, oregano, garlic. Pour all the stock in the IP; scrape the browned bits off the pot and simmer the mixture. Add the browned meat and bits; stir to mix.

4. Lock the lid and close the pressure valve. Set the IP to MEAT HIGH pressure for 42 minutes. When the timer beeps, QPR and open the lid. Transfer the meat into a large plate or cutting board using tongs. Shred the meat using 2 forks; put the shredded meat to a bowl. De-fat the cooking liquid using your preferred method. Drizzle the shredded pork with some of the defatted cooking liquid to moisten; save the rest for other uses, like stews or soups. Serve the shredded meat over salad greens.

Lettuce-Wrapped Pulled Pork

Servings|8   Prep. Time|15 minutes, plus chilling   Cook Time|50-60 minutes, plus frying
Nutritional Content (per serving): Cal|528   Fat|25.2g   Protein|65.6g   Carbs|7.1g

1 head butter lettuce, washed & dried
2 carrots, spiralized or grated
2 limes, sliced into wedges
2 tablespoons vegetable oil
4 pounds (2 kilograms) pork roast (leg or shoulder)
Water

Spice blend:
2 teaspoons oregano
1/8 teaspoon coriander
1 teaspoon white pepper
1 teaspoon garlic powder
1 teaspoon cumin
1 tablespoons cocoa powder (unsweetened)
1 tablespoon salt
1 onion (large), finely chopped

1. A day before cooking, Mix all the spice blend ingredients. Slice the pork into manageable pieces. Rub the meat with the spice blend and onion. Wrap the meat with its original butcher's paper; refrigerate overnight.
2. Set the IP to SAUTE. Add the roast; cook till all the sides are brown. Add enough water to almost cover the meat, around 2 up to 3 cups. Lock the lid and close the pressure valve. Set to MANUAL HIGH pressure for 50 up to 60 minutes. When the timer beeps, press CANCEL, NPR completely, then QPR and open the lid. Transfer the pork to a serving dish. Shred the meat into strips using 2 forks.

3. Set the IP to SAUTÉ. Cook the cooking juices till reduced by 1/2 and de-fat using your preferred method. Put the oil in a sauté pan (large). When hot, add the shredded pork; cook till light brown. Drizzle with some of the cooking liquid to add some spice.

4. To assemble: Put shredded meat into a lettuce cup; top with carrots. Drizzle with fresh squeezed lime juice.

Zuppa Toscana

Servings|6   Prep. Time|25 minutes   Cook Time|25-30 minutes
Nutritional Content (per serving): Cal|514   Fat|37g   Protein|21.6g   Carbs|22g

1 bunch kale, destemmed
1 cup coconut milk
1 pound ground Italian sausage
1 teaspoon black pepper (fresh ground)
1 teaspoon salt
1 yellow onion (medium), diced
2 cloves garlic, minced

3 teaspoons Italian parsley (fresh), with extra to garnish
4 white sweet potatoes (large), peeled & diced
5 cups bone broth (chicken)
6-7 slices bacon, chopped

1. Set the IP to SAUTE. Add the bacon; cook till crisp. Transfer to a plate; leave the grease in the pot. Put the onion in the pot; saute for 5 up to 6 minutes or till translucent. Add the garlic; saute for 3 up to 4 minutes or till fragrant. Add the sausage; saute till cooked through. If desired, remove some of the fat.

2. Press CANCEL. Add the broth, milk, pepper, salt, and sweet potato; stir to mix. Lock the lid and close the pressure valve. Set to HIGH pressure for 13 minutes. When the timer beeps, press CANCEL, NPR completely, then QPR and open the lid. Add the kale and parsley; let wilt. Serve topped with the bacon and parsley.

Turmeric Chicken & Avocado Salad

Servings|4-6   Prep. Time|15 minutes   Cook Time|12 minutes
Nutritional Content (per serving): Cal|437   Fat|26.9g   Protein|39.8g   Carbs|9g

4 cups bone broth (chicken)
2 teaspoons turmeric powder
2 green onions, sliced
1/4 cup packed parsley or cilantro (fresh), chopped
1/2 teaspoon sea salt (pink Himalayan)
1/2 teaspoon onion powder

1/2 teaspoon garlic powder
1/2 cup coconut cream (without fillers, preservatives, etc.)
1 ripe avocado (large)
1 pound chicken breasts, cooked & shredded
1 lemon (small), juice only

1. Put the chicken in your IP. Add 4 cups of broth or enough to cover the meat. Add preferred seasoning, such as pepper, salt, onion powder, garlic powder, and herbs. Lock the lid and close

the pressure valve. Set to MEAT/STEW for 12 minutes. When the timer beeps, QPR and open the lid. At this point, you can use the chicken in any dishes. Strain the cooking broth. Store in large mason jars and refrigerate or freeze to use for other dishes.

2. Put the meat in a cutting board. Shred using 2 forks. Store in the fridge if not making right away. If serving, then continue with the recipe.

3. Put the onion powder, salt, turmeric powder, garlic powder, coconut cream, lemon juice, and avocado in a food processor; process till soft and creamy. Mix the shredded chicken with the avocado cream; stir in the cilantro and parsley. Serve. You can refrigerate leftovers for 3-4 days maximum. Serve wrapped in lettuce leaves or with sweet potato chips.

Chicken Taquitos

Servings|4-6   Prep. Time|**10 minutes**   Cook Time|**20 minutes**
Nutritional Content (per serving): Cal|**364**   Fat|**20g**   Protein|**28g**   Carbs|**18g**

2 tablespoons parmesan cheese, grated
1/4 teaspoon sea salt
1/4 cup broth or water
1/2 cup cream cheese
1 pound chicken breasts
1 1/2 tablespoons taco seasoning, see options below

Taco seasoning option 1:
1 teaspoon cilantro
1 teaspoon garlic
1 teaspoon turmeric
1/8 teaspoon cinnamon
1/8 teaspoon cloves
2 1/2 teaspoon onion (minced dried)
3/4 teaspoon sea salt

Taco seasoning option 2:
1 teaspoon cilantro
1 teaspoon garlic
1 teaspoon oregano
1 teaspoon turmeric
1/2 teaspoon onion
2 1/2 teaspoon cumin

1. Except for the cream cheese, put the rest of your ingredients in your IP. Lock the lid and close the pressure valve. Set to HIGH pressure for 15 minutes. When the timer beeps, press CANCEL, NPR completely, then QPR and open the lid. Transfer the meat to a bowl; shred using 2 forks. Add 3/4 of the cooking juices in the bowl; discard the rest. Add the cream cheese to the bowl; stir to mix well. Serve.

Chicken Shawarma

Servings|**6**   Prep. Time|**1 hour**   Cook Time|**4 minutes**
Nutritional Content (per serving): Cal|**216**   Fat|**7g**   Protein|**33g**   Carbs|**2g**

1 teaspoon garlic powder
1 teaspoon onion powder
1/2 teaspoon pepper
1/2 teaspoon salt
1/4 teaspoon cinnamon
1/4 teaspoon turmeric

2 pounds chicken breasts/thighs (skinless & boneless)
2 tablespoons lemon juice
2 tablespoons olive oil
2 teaspoons cumin
2 teaspoons paprika

1. Mix the chicken with the rest of the ingredients. Refrigerate and marinate for at least 1 hour or overnight. Add the chicken and the marinade in your IP. Lock the lid and close the pressure valve. Set to MANUAL for 8 minutes. When the timer beeps, press CANCEL, NPR completely, then QPR and open the lid. Shred the chicken meat. Serve as desired.

SIDE DISHES

2-Ways Cauliflower Rice

Servings|4   Prep. Time|**5 minutes**   Cook Time|**15 minutes**
Nutritional Content (per serving): Cal|**78**   Fat|**7.1g**   Protein|**1.4g**   Carbs|**3.7g**

1 cup water, for the IP
1 head cauliflower (medium or large)
1/2 teaspoon parsley (dried)
1/4 teaspoon salt, or to taste
2 tablespoons olive oil

Optional seasonings:
Lime juice or lime wedges
Cilantro (fresh)
1/4 teaspoon turmeric
1/4 teaspoon paprika
1/4 teaspoon cumin

1. Wash your cauliflower; trim off the leaves. Chop the head into large pieces. Put the IP trivet and pour the water into the inner pot. Put the cauliflower on the trivet. Lock the lid and close the pressure valve. Set to MANUAL for 1 minute. When the timer beeps, QPR and open the lid.
2. Remove the trivet from the pot. Pour the water out. Return the inner pot to the housing. Set the IP to SAUTÉ. Add the oil and the cauliflower. Break the cauliflower using a potato masher right in the pot. While stirring and heating, add your desired spices. Add parsley and salt for basic cauliflower rice. Add the optional seasonings and serve with cilantro and squeeze of lime juice for cilantro-lime version. Or try your own seasonings. When the seasonings are well mixed and the cauliflower rice is a bit toasted, turn off the SAUTÉ function. Serve warm.

Steamed Broccoli

Servings|**2-3**   Prep. Time|**5 minutes**   Cook Time|**0 minutes**
Nutritional Content (per serving): Cal|**31**   Fat|**0.3g**   Protein|**2.5g**   Carbs|**6g**

1/4 cup water
2 up to 3 cups broccoli florets

Ice bath

1. Put the IP steamer basket and pour 1 cup water in the inner pot. Put the broccoli in the basket. Lock the lid and close the pressure valve. Set to MANUAL HIGH pressure for 0 minutes. When the timer beeps, QPR and open the lid. Immediately transfer the broccoli to the ice bath to stop cooking and help them keep their bright green color.

Caramelized Onions

Servings | **1 cup**   Prep. Time | **15 minutes**   Cook Time | **36 minutes**
Nutritional Content (per 1 tablespoon): Cal | **27**   Fat | **1.9g**   Protein | **0.3g**   Carbs | **2.3g**

1/2 teaspoon salt (kosher)
1/4 cup water
3 onions (large), halved & sliced into 1/8-inch chunks
3 tablespoons unsalted butter

1. Set the IP to SAUTÉ. Add the butter. When melted, add the onion; sprinkle with salt. Sauté for 8 minutes or till soft and slightly brown, stirring occasionally. Add the water. Lock the lid and close the pressure valve. Set to MANUAL HIGH pressure for 20 minutes. When the timer beeps, QPR and open the lid.
2. Set the IP to SAUTÉ again. Cook the onion for 5 up to 8 minutes or till the cooking liquid is reduced, constantly stirring. Let the caramelized onion. Store them in airtight containers and keep refrigerated for up to 1 week. Use as needed In French onion soup, frittatas, quiches, dips, pasta dishes, tarts, pizzas, deli sandwiches, burgers, salads, and more.

Baked Sweet Potatoes

Servings | **6**   Prep. Time | **15minutes**   Cook Time | **10 minutes**
Nutritional Content (per serving): Cal | **177**   Fat | **0.3g**   Protein | **2.3g**   Carbs | **41.8g**

6 sweet potatoes (medium), around 150 grams each
2 cups water, for the IP

1. Wash your potatoes clean and then prick them. Put the IP trivet and pour the water into the inner pot. Put the potatoes on the trivet. Lock the lid and close the pressure valve. Set to MANUAL HIGH pressure for 10 minutes. When the timer beeps, QPR and open the lid. Let the potatoes cool a bit and serve. Store leftovers in airtight containers and keep refrigerated for 5 days maximum.
NOTES: Set the timer to 12 up to 15 minutes if using large sweet potatoes.

Steamed Asparagus

Servings|4   Prep. Time|**20 minutes**   Cook Time|**2 minutes**
Nutritional Content (per serving): Cal|**84**   Fat|**7.1g**   Protein|**2.5g**   Carbs|**4.6g**

Pepper, for sprinkling
Mediterranean sea salt (fresh milled)
2 tablespoons olive oil
1 tablespoon onion, diced

1 pound asparagus, cleaned & snap off 1-inch of the tough, woody stalk
1 cup water

1. Put the IP trivet and pour the water into the inner pot. Put the asparagus on the rack; drizzle with the oil and sprinkle the onion on them. Lock the lid and close the pressure valve. Set to STEAM for 2 minutes. When the timer beeps, QPR and open the lid. Transfer the asparagus to a serving platter. Season with pepper and salt. Serve.

Steamed Carrot Flowers

Servings|4   Prep. Time|**5 minutes**   Cook Time|**10 minutes**
Nutritional Content (per serving): Cal|**46**   Fat|**0g**   Protein|**0.9g**   Carbs|**11.2g**

1 cup water, for the IP
1 pound thick carrots (500 grams), peeled

1. Using a sharp knife, slice 4 or 5 long grooves along the body of each carrot; save what comes off to use for stock or sauce. Slice the carrots into a round, creating flower-shaped pieces.

2. Put the IP steamer basket and pour the water into the inner pot. Put the carrot flowers in the basket. Lock the lid and close the pressure valve. Set to LOW pressure for 4 minutes. When the timer beeps, QPR and open the lid. Transfer the carrot flowers to a serving dish; serve. Serve as is or with preferred seasoning or dressing.

Garlicky Mashed Sweet Potatoes

Servings|4   Prep. Time|**15 minutes**   Cook Time|**4 minutes**
Nutritional Content (per serving): Cal|**234**   Fat|**7.8g**   Protein|**5.9g**   Carbs|**37.1g**

4 sweet potatoes (medium)
1/4 cup parsley, chopped
1/2 cup coconut milk

1 cup homemade vegetable broth
6 cloves garlic, peeled & cut into halves
Salt

1. Slice each potato into 8 up to 12 chunks. Put them in the IP. Add the garlic and broth. Lock the lid and close the pressure valve. Set to MANUAL HIGH pressure for 4 minutes. When the timer beeps, QPR and open the lid. Mash the potatoes right in the pot using a masher or hand blender. Gradually add the milk till desired consistency is achieved. Season with salt as needed. Add the parsley; stir to mix. Season with pepper if desired. Serve.

Garlicky Broccoli

Servings|**2-4**   Prep. Time|**5 minutes**   Cook Time|**12 minutes**
Nutritional Content (per serving): Cal|**134**   Fat|**7.4g**   Protein|**5.6g**   Carbs|**14.9g**

Ice bath
6 garlic cloves, minced
1/8-1/4 teaspoon salt (fine sea), or to taste
1/2 cup water

1 tablespoon oil
1 or 2 heads broccoli (around 360 grams or 0.8-pound each), sliced into florets (around 2 up to 4 cups)

1. Put the IP steamer basket and pour the water into the inner pot. Pot the broccoli in the basket. Lock the lid and close the pressure valve. Set to LOW pressure for 0 minutes. When the timer beeps, QPR and open the lid. Immediately transfer the broccoli to the ice bath to stop cooking. Drain and set aside to air dry.

2. Pour out the water from the inner pot and dry it. Set the IP to SAUTÉ. When hot, add the oil, coating the bottom of the pot. Add the garlic; sauté for 25 up to 30 seconds – do not let them burn. Add the broccoli; stir for 30 seconds. Season to taste with salt; stir for 30 seconds. Serve.

Steamed Artichokes

Servings | **2-4**   Prep. Time | **5 minutes**   Cook Time | **35 minutes**
Nutritional Content (per 2 servings): Cal | **77**   Fat | **0.2g**   Protein | **5.3g**   Carbs | **17.4g**

1 cup water, for the IP
1 lemon wedge

2 whole artichokes (whole), around 5 1/2 ounces each

1. Rinse your artichoke clean; remove any damaged outer leaves. Using a sharp knife, carefully trim the stem off and the top third from each piece. Rub the cut top with the lemon wedge to prevent them from browning. Put the IP trivet and pour the water into the inner pot.

2. Lock the lid and close the pressure valve. Set to MANUAL for 20 minutes. When the timer beeps, press CANCEL, NPR for 10 minutes, then QPR and open the lid. Remove the artichokes from the IP. Serve them with your preferred dipping, such as garlic butter.
NOTES: Set the cooking time for 15 minutes for small artichokes and for 25 minutes if using large ones.

Brussels Sprouts

Servings | **4**   Prep. Time | **5 minutes**   Cook Time | **3 minutes**
Nutritional Content (per serving): Cal | **106**   Fat | **6.2g**   Protein | **5g**   Carbs | **11.4g**

1 cup water, for the IP
1 pound Brussels sprouts
1/4 cup pine nuts

Olive oil
Pepper & salt

1. Put the IP steamer basket and pour the water into the inner pot. Put the Brussels sprouts in the basket. Lock the lid and close the pressure valve. Set to MANUAL HIGH pressure for 3 minutes. When the timer beeps, QPR and open the lid. Transfer the Brussels sprouts to a serving dish; season with the oil, pepper, and salt, then sprinkle with the pine nuts.

Cauliflower Mash

Servings|**4**   Prep. Time|**15 minutes**   Cook Time|**5 minutes**
Nutritional Content (per serving): Cal|**87**   Fat|**7.6**   Protein|**1.8g**   Carbs|**4.2g**

1 cup water, for the IP
1 head cauliflower, coarsely chopped
1/4 cup heavy cream

2 tablespoons butter
Paprika, to garnish, if desired
Pepper & salt, to taste

1. Wash your cauliflower clean; remove the cauliflower. Slice it into halves and then cut out the core at an angle. Chop into pieces, removing any core left. Put the IP steamer basket and pour the water into the inner pot. Put the cauliflower in the basket. Lock the lid and close the pressure valve. Set to MANUAL HIGH pressure for 5 minutes.
2. When the timer beeps, QPR and open the lid. Transfer the cauliflower to your food processor. Add the heavy cream, butter, and season with pepper and salt to taste. Process till desired smoothness is achieved. Sprinkle with paprika if desired.

Saag

Servings|**4**   Prep. Time|**15 minutes**   Cook Time|**15 minutes**
Nutritional Content (per serving): Cal|**152**   Fat|**7.5g**   Protein|**7.6g**   Carbs|**18.5g**

4 garlic cloves, minced
2-inch knob ginger, minced
2 teaspoons salt
2 tablespoons ghee (with extra to serve)
2 onions (medium), diced
1/2 teaspoon turmeric
1/2 teaspoon black pepper (fresh ground)

1 teaspoon garam masala
1 teaspoon cumin
1 teaspoon coriander
1 pound spinach, rinsed
1 pound mustard greens, rinsed
Pinch fenugreek leaves (dried)

1. Set the IP to SAUTÉ mode. Add the ghee. When melted, add the onion, ginger, garlic, and spices; stir-fry for 2 up to 3 minutes. Add the spinach; stir till wilted. Add the mustard greens; press CANCEL. Lock the lid and close the pressure valve. Set to POULTRY for 15 minutes.

2. When the timer beeps, QPR and open the lid. Transfer the mixture to your blender; blend till desired consistency is achieved. Return the blended mixture to the pot. Keep on KEEP WARM mode till serving. Top with 1 spoonful of ghee; serve.
NOTES: This dish tastes even better the next day. If it comes out too thin, pour some blended saag to a serving bowl; add cassava flour and mix till dissolved. Add the rest of the saag; mix well.

Turnip Greens & Bacon

Servings|4   Prep. Time|**15 minutes**   Cook Time|**30 minutes**
Nutritional Content (per serving): Cal|**192**   Fat|**10.4g**   Protein|**14.1g**   Carbs|**10.8g**

3-4 slices bacon, chopped into small pieces
2 cups chicken broth
1/2 up to 1 cup ham (smoked) necks/hocks
1/2 cup onion, diced

1 pound turnip greens (bagged)
Pepper & salt, to taste
Splash olive oil (extra-virgin)

1. Set the IP to SAUTÉ. Add a splash of olive oil. Add the onion, bacon, and ham; sprinkle with pepper and salt. Sauté till the meat is cooked and the fat is rendered. Add the broth and then the greens. Lock the lid and close the pressure valve. Set to HIGH pressure for 30 minutes. When the timer beeps, QPR and open the lid. Serve warm.

Cajun Greens

Servings|4   Prep. Time|**15 minutes**   Cook Time|**20 minutes**
Nutritional Content (per serving): Cal|**257**   Fat|**11.7g**   Protein|**22.6g**   Carbs|**15.4g**

1 onion, chopped
1 pound ham (uncured), fully cooked & chopped into large chunks
1 tablespoon bacon grease
1 turnip, chopped
1/2 cup poultry broth (use bone broth if available)

1/8 teaspoon salt
2 teaspoons (around 2 cloves) garlic, crushed
6 cups preferred raw greens (mustard, kale, collard, turnip, spinach, etc.)

1. Put everything in your IP. Lock the lid and close the pressure valve. Set to MANUAL HIGH pressure for 20 minutes. When the timer beeps, press CANCEL, NPR for 10 minutes, then QPR and open the lid. Stir the ingredients to mix them; serve.

Garlic & Lemon Kale

Servings|**4-6**   Prep. Time|**10 minutes**   Cook Time|**5 minutes**
Nutritional Content (per serving): Cal|**90**   Fat|**3.5g**   Protein|**3.5g**   Carbs|**12.7g**

3 cloves garlic, slivered
1/2 teaspoon salt (kosher)
1/2 lemon, juiced
1/2 cup water

1 tablespoon olive oil
1 pound kale, cleaned & stems trimmed
Black pepper (fresh ground)

1. Set the IP to SAUTÉ. Add the oil and garlic; stir for 2 minutes or till the garlic is fragrant. Stir in a large handful of kale in the oil mixture. Pack the remaining kale in the pot – it will be full. Do not worry, they will quickly wilt; just pack them enough to allow you to close the lid. Season with the salt; drizzle the water on top.
2. Lock the lid and close the pressure valve. Set to HIGH pressure for 5 minutes. When the timer beeps, QPR and open the lid. Squeeze the lemon juice over the kale. Stir in the black pepper. Transfer the mixture to a serving dish, leaving as much of the cooking liquid as possible. Serve.

Collard Greens & Bacon

Servings|**6-8**   Prep. Time|**5 minutes**   Cook Time|**30 minutes**
Nutritional Content (per serving): Cal|**123**   Fat|**8.4g**   Protein|**8.7g**   Carbs|**4.4g**

1/4 pound bacon, chopped into 1-inch pieces
1/2 teaspoon salt (kosher)
1/2 cup water

1 pound collard greens, cleaned & stems trimmed
Black pepper (fresh ground)

1. Spread your bacon in the bottom of your IP. Press SAUTÉ; cook them for 5 minutes or till brown and crisp, occasionally stirring. Stir in a large handful of collard green sot coat with the bacon grease; cook till slightly wilted. Pack the rest of the greens in the pot – it will be full. Do not worry, they will quickly wilt; just pack them enough to allow you to close the lid. Season with the salt; drizzle the water on top.
2. Lock the lid and close the pressure valve. Set to HIGH pressure for 20 minutes. When the timer beeps, QPR and open the lid. Pour the collard greens into a serving platter. Season with black pepper. Serve.

Braised Kale w/ Carrots

Servings|**2**   Prep. Time|**20 minutes**   Cook Time|**8 minutes**
Nutritional Content (per serving): Cal|**207**   Fat|**6.8g**   Protein|**7.3g**   Carbs|**31.8g**

1 onion (medium), thinly sliced
1 tablespoon ghee or preferred cooking fat
1/2 cup chicken broth
10 ounces kale (packaged), leaves & stems chopped roughly
3 carrots (medium), cut into 1/2-inch chunks
5 cloves garlic, peeled & roughly chopped
Aged balsamic vinegar
Pepper (fresh ground)
Salt (kosher)

1. Set the IP to SAUTÉ NORMAL mode. Add the ghee. When melted, add the carrots and onions; sauté till soft. Add the garlic; stir for 30 seconds or till fragrant. Pile the kale in the IP. Add the broth, making sure the pot has 1/3 headspace. Season with pepper and salt to taste.
2. Lock the lid and close the pressure valve. Set the IP to MANUAL HIGH pressure and wait till the pot reaches pressure. When pressure is achieved, Adjust the pressure to LOW and set for 8 minutes. When the timer beeps, QPR and open the lid. Stir the contents of the pot. Adjust seasoning as needed. Splash with balsamic vinegar. Ladle into serving bowls. Serve.

Sweet & Sour Red Cabbage

Servings|**4**   Prep. Time|**25 minutes**   Cook Time|**10 minutes**
Nutritional Content (per serving): Cal|**104**   Fat|**3.7g**   Protein|**2.2g**   Carbs|**17.5g**

1 tablespoon mild oil
1/2 cup onion, minced
4 cloves garlic, minced
1 cup applesauce
1 cup water
1 tablespoon vinegar (apple cider)
6 cups cabbage, chopped
Pepper & salt, to taste

1. Set the IP to SAUTÉ NORMAL mode. Add the oil and onion; sauté till they are transparent. Add the garlic; sauté for 1 minute. Add the rest of the ingredients. Lock the lid and close the pressure valve. Set to MANUAL HIGH pressure for 10 minutes. When the timer beeps, QPR and open the lid. Serve.

Salt & Vinegar Brussel Sprouts

Servings|**4-6**   Prep. Time|**10 minutes**   Cook Time|**30 minutes**
Nutritional Content (per serving): Cal|**175**   Fat|**14g**   Protein|**4g**   Carbs|**11g**

1 pounds Brussel Sprouts, sliced lengthwise into halves
1/2 teaspoon salt
1/4 cup avocado oil

1/4 cup vinegar (apple cider)
2 garlic cloves, crushed
Sea salt flakes, optional

1. Put the avocado oil in your IP. Set it to SAUTE. Once hot, add the Brussel sprouts with the cut-side down; sauté for 4 up to 5 minutes or till they are brown. Turn off the IP once they are browned to your desire.
2. Add the vinegar, salt, and garlic; stir to mix. Lock the lid and close the pressure valve. Set to MANUAL HIGH pressure for 4 minutes. When the timer beeps, QPR and open the lid. Serve. Sprinkle with sea salt as needed.

Cabbage

Servings|**4**   Prep. Time|**5 minutes**   Cook Time|**10 minutes**
Nutritional Content (per serving): Cal|**62**   Fat|**0.28g**   Protein|**2.6g**   Carbs|**14.5g**

2 teaspoons garlic
1/4 cup water
1/2 cup water, for the IP

1 onion (small), sliced
1 head cabbage
Pepper & salt for taste

1. Wash the cabbage head; remove the outer leaves. Slice the head into 3 or more pieces as needed to fit it your IP. Put the IP trivet and pour the IP water into the inner pot. Put the cabbage in an ovenproof dish/bowl that will fit your pot. Put the pot in the trivet. Add the water, garlic, onion, pepper, and salt in the bowl.
2. Lock the lid and close the pressure valve. Set to STEAM for 10 minutes. When the timer beeps, press CANCEL, NPR for 10 minutes, then QPR and open the lid. Serve.

Cauliflower & Mushroom Risotto

Servings|**4-6**   Prep. Time|**10 minutes**   Cook Time|**15 minutes**
Nutritional Content (per serving): Cal|**270**   Fat|**15g**   Protein|**8g**   Carbs|**32g**

1 cup bone, chicken, or vegetable broth
1 cup coconut milk (full-fat)
1 head cauliflower (medium)
1 onion (small), diced
1 pound shiitake, cremini, or white mushrooms (small), sliced
1 tablespoon ghee or coconut oil

1/2 teaspoon sea salt, or more to taste
1/4 cup parmesan cheese
2 tablespoons tapioca starch
2 tablespoons coconut aminos
3 garlic cloves, minced
Black pepper (fresh ground) to taste
Parsley, chopped, for garnish

1. Remove the leaves from the cauliflower; cut the florets off from the roots. Using a food processor or cheese grater, process or grate the cauliflower till rice-like in texture.

2. Put the cooking fat in your IP. Set to SAUTE; heat for 5 minutes – make sure to coat the bottom of the pot. Add the mushrooms, onion, and garlic; cook for 7 minutes or till the mushrooms sweated and are tender. Add the coconut aminos; stir for 5 minutes or till the veggies are brown. Turn off your IP.

3. Add the cauliflower, broth, coconut milk, parmesan cheese, and sea salt; stir to mix well. Lock the lid and close the pressure valve. Set the IP to MANUAL HIGH pressure for 2 minutes. When the timer beeps, QPR and open the lid. Sprinkle the starch over the risotto; stir till thick. Season with more salt or black pepper as needed. Serve warm; sprinkle with parsley.

Mixed Root Veggie Mash

Servings|**4**   Prep. Time|**20 minutes**   Cook Time|**10 minutes**
Nutritional Content (per serving): Cal|**928**   Fat|**28g**   Protein|**31g**   Carbs|**129g**

8 root vegetables (carrots, sweet potato, radishes, turnips, rutabaga, etc.)
1/2 cup coconut oil

1 tablespoon salt (coarse sea)
1 onion (large)
1 head garlic, peeled

1. Slice the garlic crosswise to expose the center of the cloves. Peel the thick-skinned root veggies. Slice all the root veggies into chunks. Coarsely chop the onion. Put the root veggies, garlic, and onion in your IP. Add 1/2 of the coconut oil and 1 cup water. Lock the lid and close the pressure valve. Set to MANUAL HIGH pressure for 10 minutes. When the timer beeps, press CANCEL, NPR completely, then QPR and open the lid. Sprinkle with sea salt. Add the rest of the coconut oil. Transfer the hot root veggies in your food processor using a slotted spoon; puree till smooth.

Savoy Cabbage w/ Cream Sauce a.k.a Wirsing mit Sahnesoße)

Servings|4-6   Prep. Time|10 minutes   Cook Time|9 minutes
Nutritional Content (per serving): Cal|**255**   Fat|**23.5g**   Protein|**8g**   Carbs|**7.1g**

1 cup bacon/lardons, diced
1 onion, chopped
2 cups bone broth
1 head (around 2 pounds) Savoy cabbage (medium), chopped finely
1/4 teaspoon mace or nutmeg

200 ml or 1/2 can coconut milk (around 1 cup)
1 bay leaf
Sea salt, to taste
2 tablespoons parsley flakes

1. Place your inner pot on a piece of parchment paper; trace around the pot. Cut out the shape; set aside. Put the inner pot in the housing. Set the IP to SAUTE. When hot, add the bacon and onion; sauté till the onions are light brown and translucent and the bacon is crisp.

2. Add the broth; scrape the browned bits off the pot. Stir in the bay leaf and cabbage. Cover with the parchment round. Lock the lid and close the pressure valve. Set to MANUAL for 4 minutes.

3. When the timer beeps, QPR and open the lid. Remove the parchment round. Set the IP to SAUTE. Bring the mixture to a bowl. Add the mace/nutmeg and coconut milk. Simmer for 5 minutes. Turn off the IP. Stir in the parsley just before serving.

Mashed Sweet Potato Muffin Tin

Servings|6   Prep. Time|5 minutes   Cook Time|20 minutes
Nutritional Content (per serving): Cal|**209**   Fat|**9g**   Protein|**3g**   Carbs|**28g**

1 to 2 cans (14 ounces each) coconut milk (full-fat)
1-2 tablespoon ghee melted
Baby spinach, optional, as much as you like to mix in
Coarse salt
Yams and/or sweet potatoes, similar shape and sizes

Equipment:
Silicon pliable muffin tins
Large ziplock bags

1. Scrub the yams/sweet potatoes. Put the IP steamer basket and pour 1 cup water in the inner pot. Put the yams/sweet potatoes on the basket. Leave a small gap between each piece to allow steam to circulate during cooking and try not to overfill the pot. You can slice the potatoes in half if they are too large to fit the pot.

2. Lock the lid and close the pressure valve. Set to MANUAL for 20 minutes. When the timer beeps, press CANCEL, NPR for 5 minutes, then QPR and open the lid. Let the potatoes cool enough to handle. Peel the skin away.

3. Add the coconut milk and salt. Puree right in the pot using a stick blender or in a food processor till desired consistency is achieved. Add milk as needed to thin out the mixture. If using spinach, mix in the amount you want. Scoop the potato mash into muffin tins. Store flat in your freezer till fully solid. Once frozen, pop them out from the muffin tins; transfer to ziplock bags. Keep in the freezer till serving.

4. To serve: Defrost overnight in your fridge; reheat in the microwave.

Mashed Sweet Potatoes

Servings|**4-6**   Prep. Time|**15 minutes**   Cook Time|**18 minutes**
Nutritional Content (per serving): Cal|**738**   Fat|**64g**   Protein|**5.5g**   Carbs|**42g**

2 pounds sweet potatoes, peeled & cut into 2-inch chunks
1 cup vegetable broth
2 tablespoons butter, melted
2-3 tablespoons heavy/whipping cream (or to taste)

Handful parsley (fresh), chopped finely
1-2 tablespoons chives (fresh), chopped
Salt & pepper, to taste

1. Peel the potatoes and slice them into 2-inch chunks. Put them in your IP. Add the vegetable broth. Lock the lid and close the pressure valve. Set to HIGH pressure for 8 minutes.

2. Put the butter in a microwavable bowl (small); microwave till melted.

3. When the timer beeps, QPR and open the lid. The potatoes are done when you can easily pierce them with a knife. If it meets resistance, pressure cook on HIGH for 2 minutes. When the potatoes are cooked, carefully remove the inner pot from the housing. Drain the potatoes, save the broth in a bowl in case you need to moisten the dish as needed.

4. Mash the sweet potatoes right in the inner pot on the countertop. Add the butter and 1 tablespoon cream. Mash the mixture, adding 1 tablespoon cream at a time as needed to achieve your desired texture. Add broth as needed. Season with pepper and salt. Add the chives and parsley. Serve.

Carrot & Sweet Potato Mash

Servings|8   Prep. Time|**25 minutes**   Cook Time|**5 minutes**
Nutritional Content (per serving): Cal|**121**   Fat|**3.4g**   Protein|**3g**   Carbs|**21g**

1 cup vegetable broth (low-sodium)
2 tablespoons butter
3 - 4 (around 1 1/2 pounds) sweet potatoes (medium), peeled, cut into 1-inch chunks

6 carrots (around 1 pound), peeled, cut into 1-inch slices
Coarse salt and pepper (fresh ground), to taste

1. Put the carrots and potatoes in your IP. Add the broth. Lock the lid and close the pressure valve. Set to MANUAL for 5 minutes. When the timer beeps, press CANCEL, NPR for 2 minutes, then QPR and open the lid. Drain the veggies in a colander, return them in the inner pot and set it on the countertop. Mash till mostly smooth or till desired consistency is achieved. Season with pepper and salt; stir well. Serve.

Sweet Potato & Cauliflower Mash

Servings|4-6   Prep. Time|**15 minutes**   Cook Time|**10-12 minutes**
Nutritional Content (per serving): Cal|**230**   Fat|**1.5g**   Protein|**8.4g**   Carbs|**49g**

1 pound cauliflower florets
1/2 teaspoon garlic powder
1/4 cup Greek yogurt (plain)
2 pounds sweet potatoes

3 tablespoons coconut milk
Parsley (fresh), chopped, for garnish
Pepper & salt to taste

1. Peel the potatoes; slice them into 1-inch chunks. Put the IP steamer basket and pour 1-inch of water in the inner pot. Put the potato and cauliflower in the basket. Set to STEAM for 10 up to 12 minutes, or till fork tender.
2. Drain the veggies. Put them in a bowl (large). Add the milk and mash. Stir in the yogurt, pepper, salt, and garlic powder. If the mixture is too thick, add 1 tablespoon milk at a time till desired consistency is achieved. Garnish with parsley. Serve.

Creamy Cauliflower Risotto

Servings|**4-6** Prep. Time|**0 minutes** Cook Time|**20-25 minutes**
Nutritional Content (per serving): Cal|**511** Fat|**37.3g** Protein|**21.5g** Carbs|**24.8g**

- 5 mushrooms baby Bella, grated or diced
- 4 cloves garlic, grated or diced
- 3 tablespoons olive oil (extra-virgin)
- 3 carrots, grated or diced, optional
- 2-4 tablespoons tapioca flour
- 2 egg yolks
- 1/4 cup butter
- 1/2 yellow onion (medium), grated or diced
- 1/2 cup dry white wine
- 1/2 cup coconut milk
- 1/2 cup chicken broth
- 1 teaspoon paprika
- 1 tablespoon oregano (fresh), chopped
- 1 head cauliflower, grated
- 1 cup parmesan cheese, grated
- 1 & 1/2 teaspoons salt
- 1 & 1/2 teaspoons black pepper (fresh ground)

1. You can grate the cauliflower, garlic, mushrooms, yellow onion, and carrots in your food processor using the grating attachment. Put the olive oil in the IP. Add the garlic and the veggies on top. Add the coconut milk, wine, butter, broth, paprika, pepper, salt, and oregano; stir to mix well.

2. Lock the lid and close the pressure valve. Set to MANUAL HIGH pressure for 5 minutes. When the timer beeps, QPR and open the lid. Stir in the cheeses till melted. Add the egg yolks; stir to mix. Add 2 tablespoons of starch; stir to mix, adding more starch as needed till desired consistency is achieved.

Coconut Cabbage

Servings|4   Prep. Time|**15 minutes**   Cook Time|**10 minutes**
Nutritional Content (per serving): Cal|**91**   Fat|**7.4g**   Protein|**1.2g**   Carbs|**6.4g**

1 & 1/2 teaspoons salt
1 brown onion (medium), halved & sliced
1 cabbage (medium), quartered, core removed, & sliced or shredded
1 carrot (medium), peeled & sliced
1 tablespoon coconut oil
1 tablespoon curry powder (mild)
1 tablespoon olive oil

1 tablespoon turmeric powder
1 teaspoon mustard powder or 1 tablespoon yellow mustard seeds
1/2 cup unsweetened desiccated coconut
1/3 cup water
2 cloves garlic (large), diced
2 tablespoons lemon or lime juice

1. Set the IP to SAUTE MORE mode. Add the oil and onion; season with 1/2 of the salt. Sauté for 3 up to 4 minutes or till soft. Add the garlic and spices; stir for 20 up to 30 seconds. Add the carrots, cabbage, desiccated coconut, and olive oil; stir to mix. Add the water; stir to mix. Lock the lid and close the pressure valve. Set to MANUAL HIGH pressure for 5 minutes. When the timer beeps, press CANCEL, NPR for 5 minutes, then QPR and open the lid. Serve with cauliflower rice, or as a side dish with chicken or fish.

Beet Pickles

Servings|4   Prep. Time|5 minutes   Cook Time|15 minutes
Nutritional Content (per serving): Cal|58   Fat|<1g   Protein|2.2g   Carbs|13g

1 cup water
6 medium (around 2-inch in diameter) beets
Balsamic vinegar

Black pepper (fresh ground)
Olive oil (extra-virgin)
Salt (kosher)

1. Wash the beets. Trim the roots so they are 2-inch long and the stems so they are 1/2 -inch long. If you buy beets with their greens on; save the leaves for stir-fry. Put the IP trivet and pour 1 cup water in the inner pot. Put the beets on the trivet. Lock the lid and close the pressure valve. Set to MANUAL HIGH pressure for 15 minutes. If cooking small beets set cooking time for 10 minutes and for larger beets for 20 up to 30 minutes. When the timer beeps, QPR and open the lid.

2. Pierce the beets with a sharp knife. If it pierces without resistance, they are done. Otherwise, pressure cook on HIGH for 2 up to 5 minutes more. Let the beets cool. Slice off the tops and slide the skins off. At this point, you can use the beets as needed.

3. To make the pickles, slice the beets into uniform chunks. Season with pepper and salt to taste. Generously splash with balsamic vinegar; marinate for at least 30 minutes, stirring 1-2 times in the process. Add a generous glug of olive oil just before serving.

NOTES: Cooking time for less than 2-inch diameter – 10 minutes, 2-inch- 15 minutes, 2-3-inch diameter – 20 minutes, and for greater than3-inch 25-30 minutes at HIGH pressure.

Herbed-Saffron Cauliflower Rice

Servings|4   Prep. Time|15 minutes   Cook Time|20-25 minutes
Nutritional Content (per serving): Cal|188   Fat|9g   Protein|23g   Carbs|5g

1 cup water, for the IP
1 head cauliflower (medium), cut into florets
1 tablespoon ghee
1 teaspoon lemon juice
1 teaspoon sea salt

1/2 teaspoon lemon zest
1/2 teaspoon saffron threads
2 cloves garlic, minced
2 tablespoons cilantro, chopped
2 tablespoons mint, chopped
Few grinds black peppers (fresh ground)

1. Put the IP steamer basket and pour the water into the inner pot. Put the cauliflower in the basket. Set to STEAM for 2 minutes. When the timer beeps, QPR and open the lid. Transfer the cauliflower to a mixing bowl. Remove the trivet and discard the water from the pot.

2. Set the IP to SAUTE. Add the ghee. When heated, add the cauliflower. With a potato masher, mash the cauliflower till the texture is rice-like. Add the saffron and garlic; stir to mix. Transfer to a serving bowl. Toss with the rest of the ingredients. Serve warm.

Rustic Root Vegetable Mash

Servings|**4**   Prep. Time|**5 minutes**   Cook Time|**3 minutes**
Nutritional Content (per serving): Cal|**186**   Fat|**8g**   Protein|**11.4g**   Carbs|**18g**

1 garlic clove, crushed
1 tablespoon duck fat (or fat of your choice)
1 tablespoon mint (fresh), chopped
1 teaspoon orange zest

1/2 cup water
1/2 teaspoon sea salt
2 cups carrots, peeled & chopped
2 cups parsnips, peeled & chopped

1. Put the IP steamer basket and pour the water into the inner pot.
Put the parsnips and carrots in the basket. Lock the lid and close the pressure valve. Set to MANUAL for 3 minutes. When the timer beeps, QPR and open the lid.

2. Drain well. Add the duck fat, sea salt, and garlic; coarsely mash the parsnips and carrots. Stir in the mint and orange zest. Transfer to a serving dish. Garnish with extra mint if desired.

SOUPS & STEWS

Beef Stew w/ Turnips & Carrots

Servings|4   Prep. Time|**15 minutes**   Cook Time|**60 minutes**
Nutritional Content (per serving): Cal|**330**   Fat|**12g**   Protein|**31g**   Carbs|**23g**

1 cup bone broth (homemade)
1 cup dry red wine
1 pound beef stew meat (grass-fed), chopped into 1-inch chunks
1 pound carrots, chopped into 1-inch chunks
1 pound turnips, chopped into 1-inch chunks
1 red onion (medium), chopped
1 teaspoon thyme (dried)
1/4 cup coconut aminos
1/4 cup parsley (fresh), chopped
2 tablespoons cassava flour
2 tablespoons coconut oil or bacon grease, divided
Salt

1. Season the beef with the salt. Set the IP to SAUTE. When hot, add 1 tablespoon of coconut oil. Add the beef; cook till all the sides are brown, around 8 minutes total. Transfer the beef to a plate; set aside.

2. Add the remaining coconut oil and onion; stir for 5 minutes or till soft. Stir in the flour and thyme; cook for 1 minute. Whisk in the wine to deglaze; scrape the browned bits of the pot. Add the broth, carrots, turnips, coconut aminos, and browned beef. Lock the lid and close the pressure valve. Set to MEAT/STEW and cook on preset cooking time. When the timer beeps, press CANCEL, NPR for 10 minutes, then QPR and open the lid. Ladle into serving bowls. Serve.

Chicken Soup

Servings|4   Prep. Time|**20 minutes**   Cook Time|**20 minutes**
Nutritional Content (per serving): Cal|**385**   Fat|**8g**   Protein|**66.6g**   Carbs|**7.9g**

4 up to 5 cups cold water
3 cloves garlic, crushed
2-3 pounds chicken, pastured and free roaming
2 carrots, roughly chopped
2 bay leaves
1/4 radish or turnips, chopped into 2-inch chunks
1 teaspoon black pepper (fresh ground)
1 tablespoon sea salt
1 tablespoon Italian seasoning OR an equal mixture of rosemary (dried), oregano, parsley, and thyme
1 stalk celery, roughly chopped
1 onion (medium), sliced or diced
Purple onion (thinly sliced) or scallion (finely chopped), to garnish

1. Put the veggies in your IP. Put the chicken on top and then season the meat with the herbs. Add the water. Lock the lid and close the pressure valve. Set to SOUP for 20 minutes. When the timer beeps, press CANCEL, NPR for 20 up to 30 minutes, then QPR and open the lid.

2. Transfer the meat to a large plate. Remove the meat from the bone. Reserve the bone for bone broth. Return the meat to the pot; stir to mix well. Using the back of a spoon, crush the carrots and celery against the side of the inner pot. Season as needed with pepper and salt. Garnish with scallion or onions and serve.

Sweet Potato & Carrot Soup

Servings|4-6   Prep. Time|10 minutes   Cook Time|20 minutes
Nutritional Content (per serving): Cal|230   Fat|7.4g   Protein|8.1g   Carbs|33.5g

1 onion (whole), chopped
1 quart chicken broth
1/2 teaspoon sage (ground)
1/2 teaspoon thyme
2 tablespoons butter

3 or 4 sweet potatoes (large, red), peeled & diced
3-4 cloves garlic, chopped
6 carrots, peeled & diced
Pepper & salt to taste

1. Set the IP to SAUTÉ. Add the butter, carrots, onion, and garlic; sauté till the onions are translucent. Add the potatoes, seasonings, and broth. Lock the lid and close the pressure valve. Set to MANUAL HIGH pressure for 20 minutes. When the timer beeps, QPR and open the lid. Puree the mixture till soft using an immersion blender.

Italian Soup

Servings|6   Prep. Time|10 minutes   Cook Time|10 minutes
Nutritional Content (per serving): Cal|581   Fat|35.7g   Protein|28.7g   Carbs|35.3g

1 cup heavy cream
1 1/2 quarts chicken stock/broth
1 onion, chopped
1 pound sausage (Italian), casing removed
1/4 cup water

2 cups kale (fresh), chiffonade (sliced into ribbons)
3 sweet potatoes (large), unpeeled & sliced into 1/4-inch chunks
4 garlic cloves, minced
4 slices bacon, rough chopped

1. Set the IP to SAUTÉ. When hot, add the bacon; cook till crisp. Transfer to a paper towel-lined plate to drain excess fat. Put the onions in the IP; sauté for 3 minutes. Add the sausage; sauté for 5 minutes, breaking them into pieces. Add the garlic; sauté for 1 minute. If needed, turn off the IP and drain excess fat.

2. Lock the lid and close the pressure valve. Set to MANUAL HIGH pressure for 5 minutes. When the timer beeps, press CANCEL, NPR for 10 minutes, then QPR and open the lid. Add the kale; stir till wilted. Add the cream; stir to mix. Ladle into serving bowls; top each serving with bacon.

Beef Meatball Soup

Servings | 8   Prep. Time | **30 minutes**   Cook Time | **13 minutes**
Nutritional Content (per serving): Cal | **231**   Fat | **5.5g**   Protein | **25.8g**   Carbs | **21g**

Meatballs:
1 egg
1 pounds ground beef, grass-fed
1 tablespoon gluten-free coconut aminos/tamari
1 teaspoon Celtic sea salt
1/3 cup cilantro (fresh), chopped
1/4 cup dill (fresh), chopped
1/4 yellow onion, finely chopped

Soup:
4-5 garlic cloves (fresh), minced
4 cups bone broth (chicken)
4 carrots, peeled & cut into 2-inch chunks
3/4 yellow onion, diced
3 celery, sliced
2 tablespoons dill (fresh), chopped
2 tablespoons cilantro (fresh), chopped
2 tablespoons butter or ghee
14 ounces artichoke hearts, drained & quartered
1 teaspoon thyme (dried)
1 teaspoon cumin
1 teaspoon Celtic sea salt
1 pound Dino kale, ribs removed & leaves chopped or sliced into ribbons

1. In a mixing bowl (large), mix all the meatball ingredients gently till well combined. Form the mixture into 2-inch balls; put them on a plate and set aside. Add your preferred cooking fat in the IP; set it to SAUTÉ. Add the onion, garlic, thyme, cumin, and sea salt; sauté for 6 minutes, stirring occasionally.

2. Press CANCEL. Add the carrots, artichoke hearts, kale, cilantro, dill, and broth; stir to mix. Gently add the meatballs in the pot. Lock the lid and close the pressure valve. Set to SOUP for 13 minutes. When the timer beeps, press CANCEL, NPR completely, then QPR and open the lid. Serve topped with cilantro.

Turmeric Sweet Potato Soup

Servings|8   Prep. Time|**20 minutes**   Cook Time|**20 minutes**
Nutritional Content (per serving): Cal|**117**   Fat|**4.2g**   Protein|**4g**   Carbs|**16.1g**

6 carrots, peeled & sliced
4 cups vegetable broth
4 cloves garlic, coarsely chopped
3-4 sweet potatoes, (large), peeled & diced
2 teaspoons turmeric (ground)

2 tablespoons coconut oil
1 teaspoon paprika
1 onion, (large), chopped
Pepper & salt

1. Set the IP to SAUTÉ. Add the oil, carrots, garlic, and onion; sauté till the onions are transparent. Add the potatoes, broth, pepper, salt, turmeric, and paprika. Lock the lid and close the pressure valve. Set to MANUAL HIGH pressure for 20 minutes.

2. When the timer beeps, QPR and open the lid. Puree right in the pot using an immersion blender or puree in your stand blender. Serve garnished with crisp fried shallots.

Bacon & Potato Chowder

Servings|8   Prep. Time|**5 minutes**   Cook Time|**5 minutes**
Nutritional Content (per serving): Cal|**629**   Fat|**15.3g**   Protein|**27.3g**   Carbs|**49g**

1 clove garlic, minced
1 cup heavy cream
1 onion (large), small diced
1 pound bacon, fried crisp & rough chopped
1 tablespoon seasoning salt
1 teaspoon black pepper (fresh ground)
1/2 cup coconut milk

1/4 cup butter
3 stalks celery, sliced thin
4 cups chicken stock
5 pounds sweet potatoes, peeled & cubed
Parmesan cheese (shredded), sour cream, and green onion (diced) for garnish

1. Put the potato in your IP. Add the butter, pepper, seasoning salt, celery, onion, and garlic; stir to mix. Add the bacon and stock. Lock the lid and close the pressure valve. Set to MANUAL for 5 minutes. Lock the lid and close the pressure valve.
2Crush the veggies using a potato masher till the mixture is semi-smooth; leave a couple large chunks of potato if preferred. Add the cream and milk; stir to mix. Ladle into bowls. Top each serving with cheese, sour cream, and green onions.

Beef Bourguignon

Servings | **4**   Prep. Time | **20 minutes**   Cook Time | **50 minutes**
Nutritional Content (per serving): Cal | **707**   Fat | **30.3g**   Protein | **65.1g**   Carbs | **30.1g**

5 carrots (medium), cut into sticks
2 teaspoons rock salt
2 teaspoons black pepper (fresh ground)
2 tablespoons thyme (fresh/dried)
2 tablespoons parsley, (fresh/dried)
2 sweet potato (large), white, peeled & cubed
2 cloves garlic, minced
1/2 pound bacon rashers/tips, sliced to thin strips

1/2 cup beef stock/broth
1 tablespoon stevia
1 tablespoon olive oil
1 red onion, (large), peeled & sliced
1 pound steak, flank/stewing, cut into 1 & 1/2-inch chunks
1 cup red wine

1. Set the IP to SAUTÉ. Add the oil. Pat dry the beef; season with pepper and salt. When the oil is hot, cook the meat in batches till they are brown; set aside.

2. Put the bacon in the IP. Add the onion; sauté till the onions are brown. Return the browned beef. Add the rest of the ingredients. Lock the lid and close the pressure valve. Set the IP to HIGH pressure for 30 minutes. When the timer beeps, QPR or NPR and open the lid.

Roasted Garlic Sweet Potato Soup

Servings|**15**   Prep. Time|**60 minutes**   Cook Time|**10 minutes**
Nutritional Content (per serving): Cal|**234**   Fat|**15.1g**   Protein|**8.6g**   Carbs|**17.7g**

Soup:
4 stalks celery, around 2 1/2 cups chopped
3 sweet potatoes (large), around 8 cups chunks
3 cups broth
2 cups carrots, chopped
2 cans (13.5 ounces each) coconut milk
1 teaspoon salt
1 tablespoon rosemary (fresh), chopped
1 tablespoon garlic cream, recipe below
1 pound ham, sliced into cubes
1 cup water, omit for a thicker soup

Optional toppings:
Sour cream
Parmesan cheese, shredded
Green onion
Bacon

Roasted garlic paste:
5-6 garlic heads (whole)
2 tablespoons olive oil
Salt, to taste

1. Roasted garlic cream: Put the IP steamer basket and pour 2/3 cup water in the inner pot. Slice off the top of each garlic head. Place the garlic in the basket in a single layer. Drizzle the 1 tablespoon olive oil directly on each garlic head. Lock the lid and close the pressure valve. Set to MANUAL HIGH pressure for 10 minutes. When the timer beeps, QPR and open the lid.

2. While still hot, sprinkle the top of the garlic heads with salt. When they are cool enough to handle, pinch the root area to pop out a couple of cloves at a time into a bowl (small). Mash them using a fork till they turn into a paste.

3. Soup: Put all the ingredients in your IP, omitting the water if thicker soup is preferred. Lock the lid and close the pressure valve. Set to MANUAL HIGH pressure for 10 minutes. When the timer beeps, press CANCEL, NPR completely, then QPR and open the lid. Serve topped with preferred toppings if using.

Chicken Soup

Servings | **5 quarts**   Prep. Time | **5 minutes**   Cook Time | **30 minutes**
Nutritional Content (per serving): Cal | **606**   Fat | **11.4g**   Protein | **106.7g**   Carbs | **13.1g**

8 cloves garlic, crushed
6 cups water
5 sprigs thyme, (large)
4 carrots (large), peeled & diced
2 stalks celery, diced

1-2 tablespoons sea salt
1 whole (small, around 4-5 pounds) chicken
1 white onion, peeled & diced
1 knob (golf ball-sized) ginger

1. Put the chicken in your IP. Add the thyme, ginger, celery, carrots, onion, and garlic. Add the water and season with salt. Lock the lid and close the pressure valve. Set to POULTRY for 15 minutes. When the timer beeps, QPR and open the lid.

2. Transfer the chicken to a plate (large) or cutting board; let cool slightly. With 2 forks, pull the meat from the bones into large chunks. Return to the pot; stir to mix. Serve. If desired, add some sweet potato noodles and mushrooms.

Parmesan, Sweet Potato, & Broccoli Soup

Servings | 4-6   Prep. Time | 10 minutes   Cook Time | 15 minutes
Nutritional Content (per serving): Cal | 522   Fat | 35.7g   Protein | 27.7g   Carbs | 23.8g

6 slices bacon, optional
4 cups vegetable/chicken broth, more as needed
2 tablespoons butter
2 pounds sweet potatoes, peeled & cut into small chunks
2 cloves garlic, crushed
1 cup parmesan cheese, shredded
1 cup heavy cream
1 broccoli head (medium), broken into large florets
Green onion or chives, chopped, for garnish
Pepper & salt, to taste

1. Set the IP to SAUTÉ. When hot, add the butter. When melted, add the garlic; sauté for 1 minute or till starting to brown. Add the broccoli, potatoes, and season with pepper and salt. Lock the lid and close the pressure valve. Set to HIGH pressure for 5 minutes.

2. If using bacon, cook them in your microwave or stovetop till the desired doneness is achieved. When the timer beeps, press CANCEL, NPR for 10 minutes, then QPR and open the lid.

3. Add the heavy cream and 1/2 cup parmesan cheese. Puree the mixture using an immersion blender or in a stand blender till smooth. Add more broth to thin the soup as needed; season with pepper and salt as needed. Serve topped with the remaining cheese and optional bacon if using.

Cream of Asparagus Soup

Servings|4   Prep. Time|**15 minutes**   Cook Time|**5 minutes**
Nutritional Content (per serving): Cal|**317**   Fat|**23.5g**   Protein|**13.4g**   Carbs|**16.9g**

1 lemon, organic, zested & juiced
1 teaspoon salt, or to taste
1 yellow onion, chopped
1/2 teaspoon thyme (dried)
2 garlic cloves, smashed/chopped
2 pounds asparagus (fresh), woody ends removed & cut into 1-inch pieces
3 tablespoons ghee, butter, or preferred lectin free fat
5 cups bone broth
8 ounces sour cream (organic) or coconut milk

1. Set the IP to SAUTÉ. Add the ghee. When melted, add the onion and garlic; sauté for 5 minutes or till the onions start to caramelize and the garlic is fragrant, occasionally stirring. Add the thyme; stir for 1 minute. Add the broth. Scrape the browned bits off the pot using a wooden spoon. Add the asparagus, lemon zest and juice, and zest.

2. Lock the lid and close the pressure valve. Set to MANUAL HIGH pressure for 5 minutes. When the timer beeps, press CANCEL, NPR completely, then QPR and open the lid. Puree the soup using an immersion blender or in a stand blender till smooth. While the stick blender or blender motor is running, add the sour cream and continue to puree. Return to the IP and heat as needed. Top each serving with more olive oil, sour cream, or lemon juice.

No-Noodle Turmeric Chicken Soup

Servings|4-6   Prep. Time|**30 minutes**   Cook Time|**65 minutes**
Nutritional Content (per serving): Cal|**408**   Fat|**14.6g**   Protein|**44.4g**   Carbs|**25g**

6 cups bone broth (chicken), divided
4 stalks celery, chopped
4 carrots, peeled & sliced
3-4 cloves garlic, minced
1-inch piece ginger (fresh), grated
1/2-1 teaspoon salt (fine sea), or to taste
1/2 tablespoon turmeric (ground)
1/2 sweet yellow onion (medium), diced
1 tablespoon thyme (dried)
1 tablespoon parsley (dried)
1 tablespoon oregano (dried)
1 pound chicken breasts
1 lemon (small), juice only
1 heaping tablespoon coconut oil
1 head green cabbage, (medium), shredded

1. Put the chicken in your IP. Add 4 cups of broth. Season with a bit of black pepper, salt, garlic powder, onion powder, and herbs if desired. Lock the lid and close the pressure valve. Set to MEAT/STEW for 12 minutes. When the timer beeps, QPR and open the lid.

2. Remove the chicken from the IP. Pat dry using paper towels. If preferred, shred the meat using 2 forks. At this point, you can use the cooked chicken in any recipe. Strain the broth; set aside.

3. Put the oil in a soup pot or Dutch oven, preferably large. Heat over medium-high flame/heat. When hot, reduce the flame/heat to medium. Add the onion, garlic, and ginger; sauté for 5 up to 6 minutes or till soft. Add the carrots, celery, and cabbage; stir to mix. Cook for 6 up to 8 minutes. Add the broth used to cook the chicken and the rest remaining unused broth.

4. Increase the flame/heat to medium-high and boil. Once boiling, reduce the heat to medium-low; cover and simmer for 20 minutes. Add the chicken, spices, and lemon juice. Cover and simmer for 20 up to 30 minutes. The longer you simmer it, the better the soup. Serve with cauliflower rice.

Chicken & Bacon Chowder

Servings | 6   Prep. Time | **15 minutes**   Cook Time | **30 minutes**
Nutritional Content (per serving): Cal | **885**   Fat | **64.1g**   Protein | **68.1g**   Carbs | **6.3g**

Chicken:
8 ounces cream cheese (full fat)
6 ounces mushrooms, sliced
6 chicken thighs, boneless
4 teaspoons garlic, minced
4 tablespoons butter
1 teaspoon thyme
1 cup celery-onion mix (chopped frozen)
Pepper & salt, to taste

Cooking day:
3 cups chicken broth
2 cups spinach (fresh)
1 pound bacon, cooked & chopped
1 cup heavy cream

1. Slice the chicken into chunks. Put them in a large bag (resealable). Add the rest of the chicken ingredients in bag and seal. Refrigerate till ready to cook. On cooking day, put the chicken mixture in your IP. Add the broth. Lock the lid and close the pressure valve. Set to SOUP for 30 minutes. When the timer beeps, QPR and open the lid.
2. Set the contents of the pot to mix well. Add the cream and spinach. Close the lid. Let sit for 10 minutes or till the spinach wilts with the residual heat. Scoop the chowder between serving bowls; top each with bacon.

Napa Cabbage & Pork Soup

Servings | **6**   Prep. Time | **20 minutes**   Cook Time | **25-30 minutes**
Nutritional Content (per serving): Cal | **251**   Fat | **5.3g**   Protein | **29.1g**   Carbs | **23.4g**

1 head (around 2 pounds) Napa cabbage, bok choy, or Savoy cabbage, cut crosswise into 1-inch segments
1 onion (small), diced
1 pound ground pork (chicken thighs, beef, or turkey)
1 sweet potato, (large), peeled & sliced into 1-inch chunks
1 teaspoon ghee or preferred cooking fat

2 carrots, (large), peeled & sliced into coins
2 garlic cloves, minced
3 scallions, thinly sliced
6 cups bone stock or broth
6 fresh (large) shiitake mushrooms, stemmed & thinly sliced
Black pepper (fresh ground)
Salt (kosher)

1. Set the IP to SAUTÉ. Add the ghee. When hot and shimmering, add the onion. Sprinkle with salt; sauté for 3 minutes or till softened, stirring occasionally. Add the pork; break the meat using a spatula. Stir in the mushrooms; season with salt. Cook for 5 up to 7 minutes or till the mushrooms are tender and the meat no longer pink. Stir in the garlic; stir for 30 seconds or till fragrant. Add the broth.
2. Lock the lid and close the pressure valve. Set to MANUAL HIGH pressure for 3-5 minutes. When the timer beeps, QPR and open the lid. Season as needed with pepper and salt. Ladle into serving bowls. Garnish each with scallions. Serve.

Beef & Broccoli Curry Stew

Servings | **6**   Prep. Time | **5 minutes**   Cook Time | **50 minutes**
Nutritional Content (per serving): Cal | **557**   Fat | **28.4g**   Protein | **62.9g**   Carbs | **13.7g**

2 tablespoons curry powder
2 1/2 pound beef stew chunks, or roast beef, chopped into small cubes
14 ounces coconut milk (canned)

1/2 cup chicken or water
1 tablespoon garlic powder
1 pound broccoli florets
Salt, to taste

1. Except for the milk, put the rest of the ingredients in your IP; stir to mix well while trying to keep the beef in the bottom of the pot. Lock the lid and close the pressure valve. Set to MANUAL HIGH pressure for 45 minutes. When the timer beeps, QPR and open the lid. Gently stir in the milk; stir to mix well. Season with salt as needed. Divide between serving bowls.

Loaded Cauliflower Soup

Servings | **4-6**   Prep. Time | **30 minutes**   Cook Time | **5 minutes**
Nutritional Content (per serving): Cal | **409**   Fat | **35.5g**   Protein | **16.6g**   Carbs | **7.9g**

1 cup parmesan cheese, grated
1 head (around 1/2 pound) cauliflower (large), stem & leaves removed, coarsely chopped (about 7-8 cups chopped)
1 teaspoon garlic powder
1 teaspoon salt (kosher)
1/2 cup coconut milk
1/2 onion, chopped small
2 tablespoons butter or olive oil
3 cups (24 ounces) chicken stock, with extra to thin the soup as needed
4 ounces cream cheese, sliced into cubes

For topping:
Sour cream
Parmesan cheese, grated
Green onions, thinly sliced
8-10 strips bacon, cooked crisp & crumbled

1. Set the IP to SAUTÉ. Add the butter. When melted, add the onion; sauté for 2 up to 3 minutes. Add the cauliflower, garlic powder, salt, and stock. Lock the lid and close the pressure valve. Set to MANUAL HIGH pressure for 5 minutes. While the cauliflower is cooking, prepare the rest of the ingredients. When the timer beeps, QPR and open the lid.

2. Puree the soup right in the pot using a stick blender or puree in a stand blender or food processor. Thin with broth if the mixture is too thick. If too thin, then simmer on SAUTÉ mode. Add the cream cheese and parmesan; let melt and stir to mix. Add the coconut milk; let heat through. Adjust seasoning as needed. Divide between serving bowls; top each with preferred toppings.

Fennel & Chicken Soup

Servings | **6-8**   Prep. Time | **20 minutes**   Cook Time | **30 minutes**
Nutritional Content (per serving): Cal | **181**   Fat | **6.3g**   Protein | **24.6g**   Carbs | **6g**

1 bay leaf
1 bulb fennel (large), chopped
1 cup kale or spinach, chopped
1 pound chicken breast or/and thighs (boneless & skinless), sliced into chunks
1 tablespoon oregano (dried)

1/2 onion, chopped
1/8 teaspoon salt
2 cups bone broth (chicken)
3 cloves garlic, peeled & chopped
4 cups water
4 green onions, chopped

1. Put everything in your IP. Lock the lid and close the pressure valve. Set to SOUP for 30 minutes. When the timer beeps, press CANCEL, NPR for 10 minutes, then QPR and open the lid. Divide between serving bowls; serve.

Hearty Vegetable Soup

Servings|4   Prep. Time|**15 minutes**   Cook Time|**25-30 minutes**
Nutritional Content (per serving): Cal|**332**   Fat|**14.4g**   Protein|**36g**   Carbs|**13.8g**

1 pound ground beef
1 tablespoon parsley (fresh), chopped
1/8 teaspoons black pepper (fresh ground)
1/8 teaspoons sea salt
2 cups carrot, diced

2 cups celery, diced
2 cups onion, diced
2 cups sweet potato, peeled & diced
3 cups bone stock/broth (beef)

1. Put the onion and beef in your IP. Set it to SAUTE. Cook till the beef is brown. Add the potatoes, carrots, celery, broth, pepper, and salt. Lock the lid and close the pressure valve. Set to HIGH pressure for 10 minutes. When the timer beeps, press CANCEL, NPR for 5 minutes, then QPR and open the lid. Top with parsley. Serve.

Beef Stew

Servings|**6-8**   Prep. Time|**15 minutes**   Cook Time|**80 minutes**
Nutritional Content (per serving): Cal|**286**   Fat|**8.6g**   Protein|**40g**   Carbs|**17g**

1 1/2 cups bone broth
1 1/2 cups red wine (merlot & cabernet sauvignon if desired)
1 tablespoon salt
2 dried bay leaves
2 heaping cups (around 140 grams) scallion greens and/or leek greens, chopped 2 heaping cups (around 425 grams) carrots, chopped

2 heaping cups (around 365 grams) rutabaga, chunks
2 pounds beef stew meat (grass-fed)
2 tablespoons bacon fat
4 strips bacon, sliced into small pieces
Few sprigs thyme & parsley (fresh), with extra for serving

1. Pat-dry the meat well using paper towels. Put the bacon fat in your IP. Set it to SAUTE. When melted, add the beef in batches; cook till all sides are brown. Transfer the browned meat in a bowl in the process.

2. When all the meat is browned and transferred, add the bacon & scallions/leek in the pot or till the bacon starts to crisp and the scallions/leek starts to wilt; stirring occasionally. Add the rutabaga, carrot, beef, wine, and broth; stir to mix. Tuck the herbs and bay leaf into the mixture.

3. Lock the lid and close the pressure valve. Set to MANUAL HIGH for 50 minutes. When the timer beeps, NPR completely on KEEP WARM mode, then QPR and open the lid. Sprinkle with extra herbs just before serving if desired.

Sweet Potato & Chorizo Soup

Servings|6   Prep. Time|**20 minutes**   Cook Time|**25-30 minutes**
Nutritional Content (per serving): Cal|**240**   Fat|**11.3g**   Protein|**14g**   Carbs|**22.7g**

1/4 cup butter
2 chorizo sausages (cooked), sliced into coins OR raw, casings removed
2 cloves garlic, chopped
2 leeks (large), cleaned & sliced, white parts only

3 sweet potatoes (large), peeled & sliced into 2-inch cubes
5 cups chicken or vegetable stock
Handful chopped cilantro
Juice from 1 lime
Pepper & salt

1. Set the IP to SAUTE. When hot, add the butter. When melted, add the garlic and white leeks; sauté till soft, stirring often. If using raw sausage, add them in the pot, sauté till fully cooked, breaking them in the process. If using cooked sausage, add them to the pot; cook for 1 minute then proceed. Add the sweet potatoes; stir well. Add the stock.

2. Lock the lid and close the pressure valve. Set to HIGH pressure for 6 minutes. When the timer beeps, press CANCEL, NPR completely or QPR and open the lid. Add the lime juice and cilantro. Adjust seasoning as needed. Serve.

Carrot & Leek Turmeric Soup

Servings|4   Prep. Time|**15-20 minutes**   Cook Time|**30-35 minutes**
Nutritional Content (per serving): Cal|**165**   Fat|**7g**   Protein|**6g**   Carbs|**22g**

1 teaspoon turmeric (ground)
1/2 teaspoon salt
1-2 tablespoon coconut oil
2 leeks (large), chopped
3 cups bone broth (chicken/beef)

3/4 teaspoon sage (ground)
5 cups carrots, chopped
5 spring onions, chopped
Edible flowers, to garnish, optional

1. Set the IP to SAUTE. Add the coconut oil. When melted, add the carrots; sauté for 5 up to 6 minutes or till slightly soft. Add the spring onions and leeks; lightly sauté for 1 up to 2 minutes. Press CANCEL.

2. Add the broth, spices, and herbs; stir to mix. Lock the lid and close the pressure valve. Set to MANUAL for 12 minutes. When the timer beeps, QPR and open the lid. Let cool for 10 up to 15 minutes. Using an immersion blender or high-powered blender; puree the soup till smooth. Serve topped with optional edible flowers if using and some green onions.

10-Minute Mushroom Broth

Servings|8 Prep. Time|5 minutes Cook Time|10 minutes
Nutritional Content (per serving): Cal|10 Fat|<1g Protein|<1g Carbs|2.4g

1 teaspoon (scant) sea salt (fine grain)
1/2 teaspoon pepper (freshly ground), or to taste
1-2 sprigs thyme (fresh)
15 grams or 1/2 cup porcini mushrooms (dried)
6 cloves garlic (medium), peeled & smashed
8 cups water

Mushroom-coconut version:
1/2 cup coconut milk (full-fat, add to broth

Mushroom-turmeric version:
Omit thyme, use 1/2 teaspoon turmeric instead
Couple teaspoons olive oil (extra virgin), coconut oil, or ghee

1. Mix the garlic, mushrooms, and water in your IP. Lock the lid and close the pressure valve. Set to HIGH pressure for 10 minutes. When the timer beeps, gently tap or shake the pot, QPR and open the lid. Season the broth with thyme, pepper, and salt. Do not disturb for 1 to 2 minute. Stir and taste. Add more pepper and salt as needed.

Carrot & Ginger Soup

Servings|5 Prep. Time|10 minutes Cook Time|5 minutes
Nutritional Content (per serving): Cal|298 Fat|23g Protein|4.2g Carbs|23.5g

1 cup red onion, chopped
1 teaspoon salt
13 1/2 ounces or 400ml coconut milk (canned)
2 tablespoons ginger, peeled & chopped

3 cups water
3 garlic cloves, chopped
5 cups carrots, chopped
Black pepper (fresh ground), to taste

1. Set the IP to SAUTE; let heat for 2 minutes. Put all the veggies in the pot; sauté for 5 minutes, stirring occasionally. Add the water; stir to mix. Lock the lid and close the pressure valve. Set to MANUAL for 5 minutes. When the timer beeps, press CANCEL, NPR completely, then QPR and open the lid. Add the coconut milk and salt. Let cool for 10 minutes, stirring often to help cool down. Puree the soup using a stick blender or a stand blender till smooth and creamy. Season as needed with black pepper. Serve.

Chicken & Avocado Soup

Servings|4   Prep. Time|**10 minutes**   Cook Time|**25 minutes**
Nutritional Content (per serving): Cal|**503**   Fat|**34g**   Protein|**24g**   Carbs|**22g**

1 bunch cilantro
1 bunch green onion, minced, white and green parts separated
1 teaspoon sea salt (coarse), or to taste
2 cups chicken, cooked & shredded

2 quarts chicken stock
3 avocados
3 limes, juice only
3 tablespoons olive oil (extra-virgin)
6 cloves garlic, minced

1. Set the IP to SAUTE. Add the olive oil. When hot, add the white parts of the green onion; sauté for 1 1/2 minutes or till tender. Add the garlic; stir for 30 seconds. Add the stock, salt, and chicken. Lock the lid and close the pressure valve. Set to HIGH pressure for 4 minutes. When the timer beeps, QPR and open the lid. Add the lime juice. Season as needed.

2. Peel and core your avocadoes; dice the flesh. Chop your cilantro. Just before serving, stir in the green parts of the green onions and cilantro. Top each serving with avocado.

Balsamic Beef & Cabbage Soup

Servings|6   Prep. Time|**40 minutes**   Cook Time|**40 minutes**
Nutritional Content (per serving): Cal|**366**   Fat|**22.4g**   Protein|**22.1g**   Carbs|**19.6g**

1 clove garlic, chopped
1 cup mushrooms, sliced
1 pound beef stew meat (grass-fed)
1 red onion, chopped
1 tablespoon oregano (dried)
1 tablespoon rosemary
1 teaspoon salt
1 white sweet potato, chopped into 1-inch chunks

1/2 cup balsamic vinegar
1/2 cup olive oil
2 carrots, sliced
2 cups water
2 tablespoons basil (dried)
3 cups cabbage, shredded
4 cups beef broth

1. Put the beef, vinegar, oil, garlic, and rosemary in a bowl (large) or resealable plastic bag (gallon). Mix well; refrigerate and marinate for 30 minutes.

2. Set the IP to SAUTE. Add the beef and marinade. Cook for 10 minutes; stirring often. Press CANCEL. Add the rest of the ingredients. Lock the lid and close the pressure valve. Set to SOUP for 30 minutes. When the timer beeps, QPR and open the lid. Serve.

Chicken Vegetable Soup

Servings | **2 1/2 quarts**   Prep. Time | **15 minutes**   Cook Time | **20 minutes**
Nutritional Content (per serving): Cal | **336**   Fat | **17g**   Protein | **25.3g**   Carbs | **22g**

1 1/4 pounds (around 6 large pieces) carrots, sliced
1 handful thyme (fresh)
1 pound (around 1 large piece) leeks, sliced white & green parts

1 pound chicken breasts, chopped into 1/2-inch chunks
1 pound sliced celery (about 1 large bunch)
2 quarts chicken broth
2 teaspoons sea salt
3 tablespoons olive oil (extra-virgin)

1. Set the IP to SAUTE MORE mode. Add the olive oil. When hot, add the chicken; sauté for 5 minutes, frequently stirring. Press CANCEL. Add the veggies, broth, thyme, and sea salt. Lock the lid and close the pressure valve. Set to MANUAL HIGH pressure for 15 minutes. When the timer beeps, QPR and open the lid. Adjust seasoning as needed.

Chicken Drumstick Soup

Servings | **6**   Prep. Time | **20 minutes**   Cook Time | **30 minutes**
Nutritional Content (per serving): Cal | **270**   Fat | **12g**   Protein | **26g**   Carbs | **15g**

2 ribs celery (large), sliced
2 carrots (medium), peeled & diced
2 bay leaves
1/2 teaspoon black pepper (cracked)
1 yellow onion (small), diced
1 rutabaga (medium), peeled & diced

1 quart chicken broth, or 1 quart water PLUS 1 teaspoon salt
1 parsnip (large), peeled & diced
1 1/2 pounds (around five large pieces) chicken drumsticks

1. Put all of the ingredients in the IP; adding the broth last; stir to mix well. Lock the lid and close the pressure valve. Set to SOUP and cook on preset cooking time. When the timer beeps, press CANCEL, NPR completely, then QPR and open the lid.

2. Transfer the chicken to a large plate or cutting board using tongs; let rest until cool enough to handle. Shred the meat from the bones; discard the cartilage, skin, and bones. Return the shredded meat to the pot; mix with the rest of the ingredients. Adjust as the seasoning as needed. Ladle into serving bowls. Serve.

FISH & SEAFOOD

Wild Alaskan w/ Broccoli or Cauliflower

Servings | 2-3   Prep. Time | 5 minutes   Cook Time | 5-9 minutes
Nutritional Content (per serving): Cal | 832   Fat | 17.5g   Protein | 156.2g   Carbs | 3.5g

1 cup cauliflower/broccoli
1 wild Alaskan cod (large filet big enough to feed 2-3 people)
2 tablespoons butter

Olive oil
Pepper & salt, to taste
Preferred seasoning

1. Choose a heatproof dish that will fir your IP. Put the broccoli/cauliflower on the dish. Slice the fillets into 2 or 3 portions. Put them on top of the veggie. Season the fish with pepper, salt, and preferred seasoning. Top each fillet with 1 tablespoon of butter and then drizzle with some olive oil.

2. Put the IP trivet and pour 1 cup water in the inner pot. Put the dish on the trivet. Lock the lid and close the pressure valve. Set to MANUAL HIGH pressure for 5 minutes for thawed or for 9 minutes for frozen fish. When the timer beeps, press CANCEL, NPR completely, then QPR and open the lid. Serve.

Steamed Shrimp & Asparagus

Servings | 2-4   Prep. Time | 20 minutes   Cook Time | 2 minutes
Nutritional Content (per serving): Cal | 329   Fat | 6.4g   Protein | 56.1g   Carbs | 11.1g

1 bunch (around 6 ounces) asparagus
1 pound shrimp (fresh/frozen), peeled & deveined
1 teaspoon olive oil

1/2 tablespoon Cajun seasoning, lemon juice w/ pepper & salt, or preferred seasoning

1. Put the IP trivet and pour 1 cup water in the inner pot. Arrange the asparagus in a single layer on the trivet. Put the shrimps on top of them. Drizzle the shrimps with the oil and sprinkle with the seasoning.

2. Lock the lid and close the pressure valve. Set to STEAM LOW pressure for 2 minutes frozen or for 1 minute for fresh shrimp. When the timer beeps, QPR and open the lid. Serve.

Crispy Salmon

Servings | **2**   Prep. Time | **5 minutes**   Cook Time | **10 minutes**
Nutritional Content (per serving): Cal | **356**   Fat | **25g**   Protein | **34.5g**   Carbs | **0g**

1 cup cold water
2 salmon (1-inch thick each) fillets, frozen
2 tablespoons olive oil
Pepper & salt, to taste

1. Put the IP trivet and pour 1 cup water in the inner pot. Put your salmon on the trivet. Lock the lid and close the pressure valve. Set to MANUAL LOW pressure for 1 minute. When the timer beeps, QPR and open the lid. Remove the salmon; pat them dry using paper towels.

2. Preheat a pan/skillet, preferably non-stick, over medium-high flame/heat. Grease the skins of the fillets with 1 tablespoon oil; generously season with pepper and salt. When the pan/skillet is very hot, put the salmon in with the skin side down. Cook for 1 up to 2 minutes or till the skins are crispy. Transfer the fish to serving plates. Serve with a preferred side dish.
NOTES: If you do not like the skin, then remove them after cooking in the IP. Increase frying time to 2 minutes.

Salmon & Broccoli

Servings | **1**   Prep. Time | **1 minutes**   Cook Time | **2 minutes**
Nutritional Content (per serving): Cal | **119**   Fat | **4.7g**   Protein | **15.9g**   Carbs | **4.7g**

160 ml water, for the IP
70 grams broccoli
72 grams salmon fillet
Pepper & salt

1. Put the IP steamer basket and pour the water into the inner pot. Chop the broccoli into florets. Season both the broccoli and salmon with pepper and salt. Put them in the basket. Lock the lid and close the pressure valve. Set to STEAM for 2 minutes. When the timer beeps, press CANCEL, NPR completely, then QPR and open the lid. Serve.

NOTES: If doubling this dish, then set the cooking time for 3 minutes.

Clam Chowder

Servings | **16** Prep. Time | **20 minutes** Cook Time | **25 minutes**
Nutritional Content (per serving): Cal | **152** Fat | **6.6g** Protein | **8.7g** Carbs | **15g**

1 quart bone broth (chicken)
1 tablespoon salt, or to taste
1 tablespoon whole thyme (dried)
1 teaspoon black pepper (fresh ground)
1 & 1/2 cups onion, diced
16 ounces clam juice (bottled)
2 pounds cauliflower (frozen florets)
3 cans (6.5-ounces each) whole clams, chopped
4 cloves garlic
4-5 cups celeriac root, peeled & diced into 1/4-inch chunks
8 ounces bacon, chopped

1. Set the IP to SAUTÉ. Add the bacon; cook for 5 up to 7 minutes or till almost crispy. Transfer them to a plate lined with paper towels to drain excess fat.

2. Pour the broth in the pot. Add the cauliflower. Lock the lid and close the pressure valve. Set to MANUAL HIGH pressure for 3 minutes. When the timer beeps, QPR and open the lid. Transfer the cauliflower to a blender or food processor (high-powered/speed) using a slotted spoon. Add the garlic; puree till smooth.

3. Add the onion and celeriac in the IP. Add the pepper, thyme, salt, and clam juice. Lock the lid and close the pressure valve. Set to MANUAL HIGH pressure for 5 minutes. When the timer beeps, QPR and open the lid. Add the pureed cauliflower and bacon; stir till well mixed.

4. Strain the clams in a fine mesh sieve. Rinse well and chop them roughly. Add the chopped clams in the pot. Adjust seasoning as needed. If you want to thicken the soup, add 1 up to 2 tablespoons arrowroot flour; mix till combined and thick.

Cod Chowder

Servings | **6** Prep. Time | **20 minutes** Cook Time | **20 minutes**
Nutritional Content (per serving): Cal | **474** Fat | **16.3g** Protein | **46.9g** Carbs | **32.4g**

1 cup clam juice
1 cup heavy cream
1 cup onion, chopped
1 teaspoon old bay seasoning (or more)
1/2 cup cassava flour
1/2 mushrooms, sliced
2 pounds cod or preferred white fish
2 tablespoons butter
4 cups chicken broth
4 cups sweet potatoes, peeled & diced
4-6 bacon slices, optional
Pepper & salt, to taste

1. Put the IP trivet and pour 1 cup water in the inner pot. Place the fish on the trivet. Lock the lid and close the pressure valve. Set to MANUAL HIGH pressure for 9 minutes. When the timer

beeps, QPR and open the lid. Transfer the cod to a plate (large). Cut the fish into large chunks using a knife or fork. Set aside.

2. Remove the trivet from the IP; pour the water out from the inner pot and return to the housing. Set to SAUTÉ. Add the butter, mushrooms, and onion; sauté for 2 minutes or till the veggies are soft. Add the potatoes and broth.

3. Lock the lid and close the pressure valve. Set to MANUAL HIGH pressure for 8 minutes. When the timer beeps, QPR and open the lid. Stir in the salt, pepper, seasoning, and cod.

4. Mix the clam juice and flour in a bowl till well mixed. Add the mixture to pot. Turn off the IP. Add the cream; stir to mix well. Serve topped with crumbled crisp bacon.

Salmon & Broccoli

Servings|1   Prep. Time|1 minutes   Cook Time|2 minutes
Nutritional Content (per serving): Cal|145   Fat|5.7g   Protein|17.7g   Carbs|6.5g

72 grams salmon fillet
70 grams broccoli, chopped

Pepper & salt
160 ml water

1. Put the IP steamer basket and pour the water into the inner pot. Season the salmon and broccoli with pepper and salt. Put the fish the veggie in the basket. Lock the lid and close the pressure valve. Set to STEAM for 2 minutes. When the timer beeps, press CANCEL, NPR completely, then QPR and open the lid.

Pepper-Lemon Salmon

Servings|3-4   Prep. Time|5 minutes   Cook Time|10 minutes
Nutritional Content (per serving): Cal|591   Fat|21g   Protein|92g   Carbs|7g

3 carrots, julienned
1 pound salmon filet skin on
1/2 lemon thinly sliced
1/2 teaspoon pepper or to taste
1/4 teaspoon salt or to taste

3 teaspoons ghee or preferred lectin-free cooking fat
3/4 cup water
A few sprigs parsley dill, basil, tarragon, or combination

1. Put the herbs and water in the IP. Set the trivet on the pot. With the skin-side down, put the salmon on the trivet. Drizzle the fish with 2 teaspoons of ghee and season with pepper and salt; top with the lemon slices. Lock the lid and close the pressure valve. Set to STEAM for 3 minutes. While the salmon is cooking, prepare the carrots.

2. When the timer beeps, QPR and open the lid. Transfer the salmon to a plate. Remove the trivet from the pot. Remove the herbs and discard. Add the carrots. Lock the lid and close the pressure valve. Set to MANUAL for 1 or 2 minutes. When the timer beeps, QPR and open the lid. Serve the veggies with the salmon. Add the remaining ghee to the cooking juices; stir to mix. Drizzle the salmon and veggies with a bit of the cooking sauce.

10-Minute Salmon

Servings|4   Prep. Time|**5 minutes**   Cook Time|**5 minutes**
Nutritional Content (per serving): Cal|**520**   Fat|**16g**   Protein|**45g**   Carbs|**49g**

1 bunch dill weed, fresh
1 tablespoon butter, unsalted
1/4 teaspoon black pepper (fresh ground)
1/4 teaspoon salt

3 lemons (medium)
3/4 cup water
4 fillets salmon

1. Put 3/4 cup of water and 1/4 cup of lemon juice. Set the trivet in the pot. Put the salmon on the trivet. Sprinkle the dill on the fish. Put 1 slice lemon on top of each. Lock the lid and close the pressure valve. Set to MANUAL for 5 minutes. When the timer beeps, QPR and open the lid. Serve right away with butter, lemon, dill, pepper, and salt.

Fish & Veggies

Servings|2   Prep. Time|**10 minutes**   Cook Time|**28 minutes**
Nutritional Content (per serving): Cal|**307**   Fat|**28g**   Protein|**2g**   Carbs|**12g**

1/2 onion, sliced into strips
1/4 teaspoon basil or preferred herb
1/4 teaspoon seasoned salt
2 pieces fish (3/4 pounds total or more), skinned & deboned
4 carrots, sliced into thin dials

4 tablespoons olive oil

Equipment:
Heatproof, stackable pans that will fit your IP

1. Line bottom piece of your stacked pans with parchment paper; put the carrots inside. Drizzle with 2 tablespoons oil and 1/2 of the seasoned salt and basil. Put the Set the top piece of the stacked pan on the bottom piece; line it with parchment paper. Put the fish inside. Drizzle with the remaining oil, seasoned salt, and basil. Put the lid on and secure the fastener of the pans.

2. Put the IP trivet and pour 1 1/2 cups water in the inner pot. Put the stacked pans on the trivet. Lock the lid and close the pressure valve. Set to HIGH pressure for 28 minutes. When the timer beeps, QPR and open the lid.

3. Check if the carrots and fish are cooked to desired preference. If not, pressure cook on HIGH for 2 minutes.

POULTRY

Chicken & Broccoli Alfredo

Servings | 4   Prep. Time | **15 minutes**   Cook Time | **15 minutes**
Nutritional Content (per serving): Cal | **982**   Fat | **78.2g**   Protein | **63.8g**   Carbs | **10g**

1 stick butter
1/4 cup parsley (fresh), chopped
2 cups broccoli
2 cups heavy cream
4 chicken breasts, cubed

4 cloves garlic, minced
4 leaves basil (fresh), chopped
6 ounces Parmesan cheese, grated
8 ounces shrimp (small)
8-ounce (bar) cream cheese

1. Set the IP to SAUTÉ. Add the butter. When melted, add the cream cheese; whisk till creamy. Gradually add the heavy cream and the parmesan; whisk till the cheese melted and the mixture is creamy. Add the rest of your ingredients.

2. Lock the lid and close the pressure valve. Set to MANUAL HIGH pressure for 15 minutes. When the timer beeps, QPR and open the lid. Serve.

Creamy Chicken

Servings | 4   Prep. Time | **5 minutes**   Cook Time | **10 minutes**
Nutritional Content (per serving): Cal | **606**   Fat | **27.8g**   Protein | **71.6g**   Carbs | **14.7g**

1 heaping tablespoon sugar
1 onion (small), quartered
2 1/2 tablespoons lime juice
2 pounds chicken thighs or breasts (skinless & boneless), cut into chunks
2 tablespoons curry paste (Thai red)

2 tablespoons oil
2 tablespoons salt to taste
3 cups chicken broth
3/4 cup coconut milk
Cilantro leaves

1. Set the IP to SAUTÉ. Add the onion; sauté for 10 seconds. Add the chicken; sauté till they are no longer pink. Add the curry paste; stir to mix well. Add the broth, salt, and sugar. Lock the lid and close the pressure valve. Set to MANUAL HIGH pressure for 10 minutes. When the timer beeps, QPR and open the lid.

2. Add the coconut milk and lime juice; stir to mix well. Top with the cilantro. Serve.

Turkey Breast & Gravy

Servings|6-8   Prep. Time|**8 hours, 10 minutes**   Cook Time|**45 minutes**
Nutritional Content (per serving): Cal|**408**   Fat|**17g**   Protein|**53g**   Carbs|**9g**

Turkey breast:
1 cup cauliflower florets, frozen or fresh
1 onion, diced
1/4 cup chicken broth
3 tablespoons thyme leaves (fresh)
3-pounds (skin-on) whole turkey breast, thawed
5 tablespoons ghee, divided
6 cloves garlic minced, divided
Pepper & salt (freshly ground) to taste

Brine:
1/2 cup salt
3 cloves garlic, peeled & smashed
9 cups water
Few sprigs thyme (fresh)

Gravy:
1-2 tablespoons water
4 tablespoons arrowroot powder
Coconut aminos to taste
Pepper & salt (freshly ground) to taste

1. Brine: Stir everything till the salt is fully dissolved. Pour the brine in a large food container or resealable bag. Add the turkey. Close or seal; refrigerate for at least 4 hours up to 12 hours.

2. Turkey breast: After brining, drain the turkey. Pat dry the turkey using paper towels. Keep the elastic wrap on your turkey. Using clean fingers, carefully peel the skin away from the meat, rub the butter mixture under the skin. Alternatively, put the ghee mixture on a spoon; stick it under the skin. Use your fingers to remove the ghee from the spoon and spread the ghee by rubbing the outside of the skin. Rub the outside of the skin with 1 tablespoon ghee; season with pepper and salt.

3. Set the IP to SAUTE. When hot, add 1 tablespoon ghee. Add the garlic and onions; sauté till slightly soft, stirring occasionally. Add the cauliflower and broth; stir to mix. Put the turkey on top of the cauliflower-onion mixture. Lock the lid and close the pressure valve. Set to MANUAL HIGH pressure for 28 minutes.

4. When the timer beeps, press CANCEL, NPR for 10 up to 15 minutes, then QPR and open the lid. Carefully remove the turkey breast from the pot. Cut off the elastic wrap. Preheat the broiler; broil for a couple of minutes or till the skin is brown.

5. Gravy: Using a stick blender or high-powered blender, puree the contents of the pot till very smooth. Set the IP to SAUTE. Cook the gravy on NORMAL mode. In a bowl (small), mix the arrowroot and 1 up to 2 tablespoons water till smooth. Add the mixture in the pot. Vigorously whisk to mix; let simmer till thick to desired texture. Add the coconut aminos. Add salt and pepper to taste.

6. To serve: slice the turkey. Serve with the gravy.

Zuppa Toscana

Servings | 6   Prep. Time | **10 minutes**   Cook Time | **40 minutes**
Nutritional Content (per serving): Cal | **471**   Fat | **32.2g**   Protein | **22.1g**   Carbs | **23.7g**

5 cups chicken broth
3 sweet potatoes (large), cut into 1-inch chunks
3 cloves garlic, minced
2 teaspoons basil (dried)
2 tablespoons olive oil
2 cups large curly kale leaves (fresh), chopped

1/2 cup coconut milk (full-fat) or heavy cream
1 yellow onion (medium), chopped
1 teaspoon fennel (dried)
1 pound Italian Sausage (turkey or chicken)
Pepper & salt, to taste

1. Set the IP to SAUTÉ. When hot, add the oil and onion; sauté for 2 up to 3 minutes. Add the garlic and sausage; cook for 5 minutes or till the sausage is brown. Press CANCEL. Add the broth, potatoes, and herbs in the pot. Lock the lid and close the pressure valve. Set the IP to MANUAL HIGH pressure for 12 minutes.

2. When the timer beeps, QPR and open the lid. Set the IP to SAUTÉ/ Stir in the kale till they start to wilt. Stir in the coconut milk/heavy cream. Season as needed with pepper and salt.

Chicken 2-Ways

Servings | 4   Prep. Time | **5 minutes**   Cook Time | **15 minutes**
Nutritional Content (per serving): Cal | **180**   Fat | **0g**   Protein | **33.4g**   Carbs | **2g**

1 pound frozen chicken breasts, (skinless & boneless)
Preferred flavorful cooking liquid, see options below

Flavorful cooking liquid options:
Lemon Garlic Herb:
1/2 cup water
1/2 of a lemon juice
2 cloves garlic, minced
1/2 teaspoon basil (dried)
Pepper & salt

Thai Curry:
1 cup coconut milk (canned)
1-2 tablespoon preferred Thai curry paste (undiluted)

1. In a bowl (small) or measuring cup, mix your choice of flavorful cooking liquid. Put the chicken in the IP. Add the liquid, pouring it over the chicken. Lock the lid and close the pressure valve.

Set to POULTRY for 15 minutes for standard 4-8 ounces pieces or for 30 minutes for extra-large ones, around 1 pound each piece. When the timer beeps, QPR and open the lid.

2. Transfer the chicken to a large plate or cutting board. Shred into bite-sized pieces using 2 forks. While shredding the meat, set the IP to SAUTÉ and cook the sauce to reduce and thicken if too thin. Once thick to preference, return the shredded chicken to the pot; toss to coat with the sauce.

30-Minute Fall-Off-The-Bone Chicken

Servings | 10   Prep. Time | 10 minutes   Cook Time | 35 minutes
Nutritional Content (per serving): Cal | 297   Fat | 7.2g   Protein | 53.5g   Carbs | 1.1g

1 1/2 cups bone broth (chicken)
1 tablespoon coconut oil (virgin)
1 teaspoon paprika
1 teaspoon thyme (dried)
1 whole (around 4 pounds) chicken

1/2 teaspoon sea salt
1/4 teaspoon black pepper (fresh ground)
2 tablespoons lemon juice (fresh squeezed)
6 cloves garlic, peeled

1. In a bowl (small), mix the thyme, paprika, salt, and pepper. Rub the outside of your chicken with the spice mixture. Set the IP to SAUTÉ. Add the oil. When hot and shimmering, add the chicken breast with the breast side down. Cook for 6 up to 7 minutes. Rotate the chicken. Add the broth, lemon juice, and garlic cloves.

2. Lock the lid and close the pressure valve. Set to MANUAL HIGH pressure for 25 minutes. When the timer beeps, press CANCEL, NPR completely, then QPR and open the lid. Transfer the chicken to a serving platter; let stand for 5 minutes. Carve and serve.

Crack Chicken

Servings | 4   Prep. Time | 10 minutes   Cook Time | 25 minutes
Nutritional Content (per serving): Cal | 834   Fat | 48g   Protein | 87.8g   Carbs | 8.2g

1 cup water
2 pounds chicken breast (boneless)
2 tablespoons ranch seasoning
3 tablespoons tapioca starch

4 ounces parmesan cheese
6-8 bacon slices, cooked
8 ounces cream cheese

1. Put the chicken and cream cheese in your IP. Season with the ranch seasoning. Add the water. Lock the lid and close the pressure valve. Set to MANUAL HIGH pressure for 25 minutes. Lock the lid and close the pressure valve. Transfer the chicken to a cutting board or large plate. Shred the meat.

2. Set the IP to SAUTÉ LESS mode. Whisk in the tapioca starch. Add the parmesan cheese and shredded meat. Stir in the bacon. Serve.

Turkey Drumsticks

Servings | 6   Prep. Time | **5 minutes**   Cook Time | **40 minutes**
Nutritional Content (per serving): Cal | **209**   Fat | **5.7g**   Protein | **34.6g**   Carbs | **3g**

1 tablespoon salt (kosher)
1 teaspoon black pepper (fresh ground)
1/2 cup coconut aminos or tamari
1/2 cup water, for the IP
1/2 teaspoon garlic powder
2 packed tight teaspoons stevia
6 turkey drumsticks

1. In a bowl (small), mix the salt, stevia, pepper, and garlic powder, breaking any clumps. Season the turkey with the seasoning mixture. Pour the water and coconut aminos in the IP. Add the seasoned turkey. Lock the lid and close the pressure valve. Set to MANUAL HIGH pressure for 25 minutes.

2. When the timer beeps, press CANCEL, NPR for 15 minutes, then QPR and open the lid. Transfer the turkey to a serving dish very carefully – they will be fall-off-the-bone tender. Serve the cooking liquid as a sauce to pass at the table. If preferred, de-fat the cooking liquid before serving.

NOTES: If you prefer crisp turkey skin, brush the cooked drumsticks with some of the cooking liquid; broil till brown. The cooking liquid is also great with baked sweet potatoes.

Chicken Wings

Servings | **4-6**   Prep. Time | **5 minutes**   Cook Time | **14-15 minutes**
Nutritional Content (per serving): Cal | **786**   Fat | **38.9g**   Protein | **100.8g**   Carbs | **2.8g**

1/2 cup chicken broth or water
2 tablespoons olive oil
2-3 pounds chicken wings (I used 3 pounds)
2-3 tablespoons preferred seasonings (stay basic with salt, pepper, & garlic)
Lectin-free sauce, for serving

1. Wash the chicken clean and then pat dry. Put them in a mixing bowl (large). Add your preferred seasoning and the oil; rub the wings well till coated with the seasoning and oil and work the flavors in the meat. Put the wings in your IP. Add the broth/water.

2. Lock the lid and close the pressure valve. Set to MANUAL HIGH pressure for 9 minutes. When the timer beeps, QPR and open the lid. Carefully transfer the chicken wings to a sheet pan. Set your oven to broil; broil the chicken for 5 up to 6 minutes or till the skins are crisp, flipping halfway through cooking. Toss with preferred sauce. Serve.

Creamy Chicken & Mushroom

Servings | **4**   Prep. Time | **15 minutes**   Cook Time | **20 minutes**
Nutritional Content (per serving): Cal | **713**   Fat | **41.1g**   Protein | **72.7g**   Carbs | **14.8g**

1 can coconut cream
1 tablespoon water
1 teaspoon garlic powder
1 teaspoon onion powder
1 teaspoon salt
1 teaspoon thyme (dried)
16 ounces mushrooms (baby portabella), sliced

2 pounds chicken thighs
2 tablespoons tapioca starch
Chicken broth, as needed to fill the can of coconut cream after the content is poured out

1. The evening before cooking, refrigerate the can of coconut cream to chill overnight. Just before cooking, take the can from your fridge; do not shake or turn upside down. Open the can – the water and the cream should have separated with the coconut water on top. Pour or scoop out the coconut water from the can.

2. Add broth to replace the coconut water, filling the can to the top. Pour all the contents of the can in a bowl (medium). Add the spices; whisk till combined. Put the chicken in the IP. Put the mushrooms on top of the chicken to cover the meat. Pour the coconut cream mixture over your chicken and then add the mushrooms.

3. Lock the lid and close the pressure valve. Set to MANUAL HIGH pressure for 8 up to 10 minutes. When the timer beeps, press CANCEL, NPR completely, then QPR and open the lid. Transfer the mushrooms and chicken to a serving platter using a slotted spoon, leaving as much of the cooking liquid in the IP.

4. Scoop out 1/2 of the cooking liquid and discard. Set the IP to SAUTÉ and boil the remaining liquid. In a bowl (small), whisk the starch and water till smooth. When the cooking liquid is boiling; whisk in the starch mixture. mix till the cooking liquid is smooth and thick like gravy. Turn off your IP. Ladle the gravy over the chicken and mushrooms. Serve.

Pesto Chicken w/ Carrots & Sweet Potatoes

Servings | **4**   Prep. Time | **30 minutes**   Cook Time | **11 minutes**
Nutritional Content (per serving): Cal | **794**   Fat | **21.2g**   Protein | **104.7g**   Carbs | **41.5g**

1 piece (6 to 8 ounces) onion, peeled & cut vertically into 1/2-inch slices
1 pound baby carrots

1/2 cup chicken stock
1/2 tablespoon olive oil (extra-virgin)
1/3 cup pesto (prepared)

3 pounds chicken thighs (bone in), skins removed, visible fat trimmed

8 pieces (2-inch) sweet potatoes (around 1 1/2 pounds), scrubbed & peeled

1. Toss the chicken with the oil to coat well. Set the IP to SAUTÉ. When hot, add 4 pieces chicken; cook for 3 minutes each side or till all sides are brown. Transfer the browned chicken to a bowl. Cook the rest of the chicken till brown. Turn off your IP.

2. Add the pesto in the bowl with the browned chicken; toss to coat. Pour the stock in the IP. Add the onions. Set a trivet in the pot. Put the pesto coated chicken on the trivet. Add the carrots and potatoes on top of the meat.

3. Lock the lid and close the pressure valve. Set the IP to MANUAL HIGH for 11 minutes. When the timer beeps, QPR and open the lid. Transfer the meat and veggies to a serving dish using a slotted spoon. De-fat the cooking liquid. Serve the chicken and vegetables with the defatted sauce on the side.

Chicken w/ Sweet Potatoes & Mixed Veggies

Servings|8   Prep. Time|5 minutes   Cook Time|25 minutes
Nutritional Content (per serving): Cal|506   Fat|30.7g   Protein|23.9g   Carbs|33.5g

3 cups chicken broth
2 tablespoons tapioca starch
2 cups sweet potatoes, chunked
16 ounces parmesan cheese

16 ounces mixed veggies (bagged frozen)
1 pound chicken breast
1 onion, small diced
1 cup heavy cream

1. Put the chicken chunks in your IP. Add the potatoes and veggies. Add the broth. Lock the lid and close the pressure valve. Set to MANUAL HIGH pressure for 14 minutes. When the timer beeps, QPR and open the lid. Set the IP to SAUTÉ. Whisk in the heavy cream and starch, and boil. Stir in the parmesan cheese and boil till thickened. Serve.

Turkey & Sweet Potato White Chili

Servings|5-6   Prep. Time|10 minutes   Cook Time|30 minutes
Nutritional Content (per serving): Cal|617   Fat|36.9g   Protein|34.4g   Carbs|43g

Soup base:
4 cups large chunks (3 medium) white sweet potatoes
3 cups bone broth, more to taste
2 cups leek whites, chopped
1 teaspoon white pepper
1 teaspoon salt

1 tablespoon bacon fat
1 cup coconut cream
Pinch nutmeg

For the turkey:
1/2 teaspoon garlic (ground)
1/2 teaspoon mustard
1/2 teaspoon salt
1/4 cup leek greens, minced, sliced till
1-2 pounds ground turkey

4 slices bacon, sliced to 1/4 -inch pieces

Crisp potato skins:
Sweet potato peels
1/4 cup coconut oil

1. Peel the potatoes; set the skins aside – do not throw them away. Set the IP to SAUTE. When hot, add the bacon; cook till crispy. Meanwhile, slice the white parts of the leek till you reach the green part. Transfer the crisped bacon to a plate.

2. Put the white leeks in the pot; sauté till starting to brown. Add the potato and broth; season with the salt, white pepper, and nutmeg. Lock the lid and close the pressure valve. Set to STEAM and for preset cooking time.

3. Meanwhile, put the turkey in a bowl. Add the salt, mustard, and garlic; set aside. Wash the green leeks part and mince; set aside. Put the coconut oil in a pan/skillet. Prepare a plate lined with paper towel; place it near the stove. Test the oil by touching it with a wooden spoon. When it sizzles, add 1 handful of potato skins; cook for 30 up to 45 seconds or till they are golden brown. Immediately transfer them to the prepared plate. Repeat the process with the rest of the potato skins.

4. When the timer beeps, QPR and open the lid. Carefully transfer the contents of the IP to a blender. Return the inner pot to the housing. Set to SAUTE. Add the turkey mixture and green leeks; saute for 5 minutes or till the meat is brown; crumbling the meat in the process and stirring often.

5. While the meat is cooking, blend the contents of the blender till smooth. Add the cream to the mixture; blend again. When the turkey is brown, add the blended puree and bring to a simmer. At this point, you can thin the soup if as desired or enjoy it thick. Stir in the crisped bacon, saving a couple pieces as topping. Scoop the soup between serving bowls. Garnish with bacon, crisped potato skin, and green onion.

Very Simple Whole Chicken

Servings|4-6   Prep. Time|15 minutes   Cook Time|14-20 minutes
Nutritional Content (per serving): Cal|676   Fat|28.6g   Protein|98.4g   Carbs|0g

1 cup water
1 tablespoons coconut oil

1 whole chicken
Preferred seasonings

1. Put the IP trivet and pour the water into the inner pot. Put the oil in a pan/skillet (large). Season the chicken with your preferred seasonings. Put the chicken in the pan/skillet; cook each side for 1 minute to sear the skin. When done, transfer the chicken to the trivet in the IP.

2. Lock the lid and close the pressure valve. Set to MANUAL HIGH pressure for 6 minutes per 1 pound of chicken, then add 2 minutes to the total cooking time. When the timer beeps, press CANCEL, NPR completely, then QPR and open the lid. You can leave the chicken in the pot longer than 15 minutes, but do not leave for more than 15 minutes. Serve. Save the bones to make your broths.

Roasted Whole Chicken

Servings|8   Prep. Time|**5 minutes**   Cook Time|**55 minutes**
Nutritional Content (per serving): Cal|**446**   Fat|**18.5g**   Protein|**65.6g**   Carbs|**0g**

1 tablespoon coconut oil
4 pounds whole chicken
Lemon pepper seasoning or preferred seasoning

Pepper
Salt

1. Set the IP to SAUTE. Add the oil. When hot, add the chicken with the breast-side down; cook till brown. Move the chicken a few times to brown the sides of the breasts as well. Flip the chicken; sprinkle with the seasonings. Lock the lid and close the pressure valve. Set to POULTRY HIGH pressure for 20 minutes. When the timer beeps, QPR and open the lid.

2. Flip the chicken. Lock the lid and close the pressure valve. Set to POULTRY HIGH pressure for 15 minutes. When the timer beeps, QPR and open the lid. At this point, the chicken should be cooked through. If not, then pressure cook on HIGH for 5 minutes more. Transfer to a serving dish. Serve.

NOTES: The meat juices will cook the meat. However, if your IP will not reach pressure, then add a splash of water. If you want to crisp the skin, broil for 5 minutes. You can also use a kitchen torch to crisp the skin.

Coconut Chicken & Sweet Potato Curry

Servings|4   Prep. Time|**10 minutes**   Cook Time|**25 minutes**
Nutritional Content (per serving): Cal|**251**   Fat|**7.7g**   Protein|**4.1g**   Carbs|**22.7g**

1 onion, finely chopped

1 small (around 250 grams/9 ounces) sweet potato

1 teaspoon ginger (ground)
1 teaspoon turmeric
2 carrots, chopped fined
2 teaspoons coriander
2 teaspoons cumin
200ml/7 fluid ounces chicken stock

200ml/7 fluid ounces light coconut milk
4 cloves garlic, crushed & chopped
8 chicken thighs (all visible fat removed)
Coriander (fresh), chopped
Spray oil (olive oil)

1. Pierce the sweet potato using a fork; microwave for 5 minutes. It should feel soft to touch. Set aside; let cool. Set the IP to SAUTE. Grease it with the spray oil. Add the carrot, ginger, garlic, and onion; fry till soft. Slice the sweet potato lengthwise into halves. Scoop the flesh into the instant pot. Add the spices. Mix well, mashing the potato roughly. Add the chicken, stock, and coconut milk. Lock the lid and close the pressure valve. Set to POULTRY HIGH pressure for 15 minutes. When the timer beeps, press CANCEL, NPR completely, then QPR and open the lid. Slightly shred the chicken into the sauce. Sprinkle with fresh coriander. Serve with preferred sides.

Coconut Basil Chicken Curry

Servings|3-4   Prep. Time|**10 minutes**   Cook Time|**35-40 minutes**
Nutritional Content (per serving): Cal|**695**   Fat|**54g**   Protein|**40g**   Carbs|**12g**

1 1/2 tablespoons curry powder (hot yellow or regular)
1 1/2 teaspoons basil (dried)
1 1/2 up to 2 pounds chicken thighs (organic)
1 red onion, diced

1 tablespoon garlic, minced
1-2 tablespoon olive oil (extra-virgin)
1-2 tablespoon tapioca starch & hot water, to thicken
2 cans coconut milk (full-fall)
2 teaspoons sea salt or to taste

1. Put the olive oil in your IP. Set to SAUTE. Season the chicken with salt. Add to the pot; cook till all the sides are brown. Transfer the chicken to a dish. Add the coconut milk, curry powder, and basil in the pot; stir to mix.

2. Return the chicken to the pot. Add the garlic and onion; stir to mix. Lock the lid and close the pressure valve. Set to MANUAL for 10 up to 12 minutes. When the timer beeps, QPR and open the lid. Shred the chicken using a fork. Mix the tapioca with some hot water to make a slurry. Add to the pot 1 tablespoon at a time; stir to mix. Serve with lectin-free salad or greens of choice.

Lemon Chicken

Servings | 5   Prep. Time | **5 minutes**   Cook Time | **90 minutes**
Nutritional Content (per serving): Cal | **509**   Fat | **35g**   Protein | **43g**   Carbs | **5g**

1 teaspoon black pepper (fresh ground)
1 teaspoon parsley (dried)
1 teaspoon salt

1 whole chicken, frozen or thawed
Juice of 3 lemons
1 cup broth or water

1. Put the chicken in your IP. Add the broth/water. Lock the lid and close the pressure valve. Set to HIGH pressure for 30 minutes for fresh or for 75 minutes for frozen meat. When the timer beeps, press CANCEL, NPR completely, then QPR and open the lid.

2. Transfer the chicken to a sheet pan; drizzle all over with the lemon juice. Broil for 5 up to 7 minutes or till the skin is golden and crisp. Remove from the oven; let rest for 10 minutes. Slice and serve.

Turkey Breast Roast

Servings | 6-8   Prep. Time | **20 minutes**   Cook Time | **30 minutes**
Nutritional Content (per serving): Cal | **426**   Fat | **14g**   Protein | **71g**   Carbs | **0g**

2 tablespoon seasoned salt
2 tablespoon infused oil (roasted garlic), for the turkey

1 turkey breast roast (boneless)
2 tablespoon infused oil (roasted garlic), for the IP

1. Coat the turkey with the oil and then rub with the seasoned salt. Set the IP to SAUTE. When the pot is hot, add the oil. Add the turkey and cook till all the sides of the meat is brown. Transfer the roast to a plate.

2. Pour 1 1/2 cups water in the inner pot; scrape off the browned bits on the pot. Carefully set the IP trivet. Put the roast on the trivet. Lock the lid and close the pressure valve. Set to MANUAL for 30 minutes. When the timer beeps, press CANCEL, NPR completely, then QPR and open the lid. Serve!

Chicken Legs W/ Lemon & Garlic

Servings|4   Prep. Time|5 minutes   Cook Time|25 minutes
Nutritional Content (per serving): Cal|149   Fat|5g   Protein|22.2g   Carbs|3g

1 cup water
1 frozen package chicken legs
1 lemon, quartered
1 teaspoon Italian herbs seasoning

1 teaspoon salt
1/4 teaspoon pepper
8 garlic cloves, peeled

1. Put the water and garlic in your IP. Add the chicken; season with the pepper, salt, and seasoning. Put the lemon on top of the meat. Lock the lid and close the pressure valve. Set to MANUAL for 25 minutes. When the timer beeps, QPR and open the lid. Serve.

Thai Chicken

Servings|4-6   Prep. Time|15 minutes   Cook Time|30-35 minutes
Nutritional Content (per serving): Cal|336   Fat|20.4g   Protein|32.3g   Carbs|4.41g

1 red onion (medium), thickly sliced
1 teaspoon Celtic sea salt
1/2 cup bone broth (chicken)
1/2 teaspoon curry powder
1/2cup coconut milk (full-fat)
1/4 cup coconut aminos or tamari
15 mint leaves (small)
1-inch ginger chunk (fresh), finely minced or grated

2 chicken breasts, diced
2 tablespoons butter, ghee, or avocado oil
4 garlic cloves (fresh), finely minced or grated
5-inch lemongrass stems, ends removed & halved
Zest and juice of 1 lime

1. Set the IP to SAUTE. Add the butter, onion, ginger, and garlic; sauté for 5 minutes, occasionally stirring. Add the chicken, cook for 2 up to 3 minutes or till no longer pink, stirring occasionally. Press CANCEL.

2. Add the broth, coconut milk, coconut aminos, curry powder, mint leaves, lemongrass, lime zest, and lime juice; stir to mix. Lock the lid and close the pressure valve. Set to POULTRY for 10 minutes. When the timer beeps, QPR and open the lid. Serve. Garnish with lime wedges and cilantro. Serve with cauliflower rice.

Lemon & Coconut Chicken Curry

Servings|6   Prep. Time|5 minutes   Cook Time|35 minutes
Nutritional Content (per serving): Cal|806   Fat|64g   Protein|51.5g   Carbs|4.3g

4 pounds chicken thighs and/or breasts
1/4 cup lemon juice
1/2-1 teaspoon lemon zest
1/2 teaspoon salt

1 teaspoon turmeric
1 tablespoon curry powder
1 can coconut milk (full-fat)

1. Mix the spices, lemon juice, and coconut milk in a glass measuring cup or bowl. Pour a little bit of the mixture in the IP. Add the chicken. Pour the rest of the coconut mixture on top of the meat. Lock the lid and close the pressure valve. Set to POULTRY HIGH pressure for 15 minutes for fresh or for 25 minutes for frozen chicken. When the timer beeps, QPR and open the lid.

2. Slice the chicken and check of the center is no longer pink. If it is still undercooked, pressure cook on MANUAL HIGH pressure for 5 up to 10 minutes more. If the chicken is cooked through, shred the meat right in the pot or transfer to a plate for shredding. Add optional lemon zest if using. Serve with roasted or steamed lectin free veggies or over cauliflower rice.

NOTES: If you want a thick soup, add 1-2 tablespoons arrowroot starch after the chicken is cooked through.

Duck Confit

Servings|4   Prep. Time|24 hours   Cook Time|2 hours
Nutritional Content (per serving): Cal|205   Fat|10.5g   Protein|24.9g   Carbs|1.24g

1 tablespoon salt (kosher)
2 bay leaves, torn into halves
4 pieces duck legs (thighs & drumsticks)
1/4 teaspoon black peppercorns (fresh ground), lightly crushed

4 garlic cloves, smashed
1/4 teaspoon allspice berries, crushed lightly
4 sprigs thyme (fresh)

1. Line a plate or rimmed sheet pan with some paper towels. Mix the allspice, peppercorns, bay leaves, garlic, thyme, and salt in a bowl (large). Add your duck legs; toss to coat well with the spice mixture. In a single layer, put the duck in the prepared sheet pan/plate; refrigerate without cover for a minimum of 24 hours up to three (3) days.

2. Brush off the thyme sprigs and garlic off the duck; reserve them. Set the IP to SAUTE. With the skin-side down, arrange the duck legs in your pot with the flesh in contact with the pot bottom as much as possible. Cook for 5 up to 10 minutes or till golden brown and the fat begins to

render. Flip the duck; cook for 5 up to ten (10) minutes more. Scatter the reserved thyme and garlic over the duck.

3. Lock the lid and close the pressure valve. Set for forty (40) minutes on HIGH pressure. When the timer beeps, press CANCEL, NPR completely, then QPR and open the lid. Let the poultry cool completely. Store it with covered with its own fat and cooking juices in the fridge. As the dark brown sauce cools, the duck fat will separate; save this for soups, sauces, or any dish needing concentrated poultry or meat stock.

4. When ready to serve; preheat your broiler. Remove the fat off the duck legs. Put them to a sheet pan with rim; broil for 3 up to five (5) minutes or till the skin is crisp. Or crisp the skin in a dry, hot pan/skillet.

Chicken & Mushroom

Servings|6   Prep. Time|5 minutes   Cook Time|30 minutes
Nutritional Content (per serving): Cal|456   Fat|37g   Protein|26g   Carbs|4.6g

1/2 teaspoon nutmeg (ground)
1 bay leaf
1 onion (large), diced
1 teaspoon black pepper (fresh ground)
1 teaspoon garlic powder
1/2 cup coconut cream, divided
2 cloves garlic, minced
2 cups cremini or baby Bella mushrooms, sliced

2 pounds chicken thighs (skinless & boneless)
2 sprigs rosemary
2 tablespoons avocado oil
2 tablespoons vinegar (red wine)
2 teaspoons fine salt

1. Preheat your IP on SAUTE mode. Add the oil, garlic, onion, and bay leaf; saute for 8 up to 10 minutes or till tender. Add the mushrooms and rosemary; saute for 5 minutes or till tender and brown. Add the chicken and seasonings; saute till the chicken is mostly brown; stirring occasionally. Add the vinegar to deglaze, scrape the browned bits off the pot. Add 1/4 cup of coconut cream. Press CANCEL. Lock the lid and close the pressure valve. Set to HIGH pressure for 10 minutes. When the timer beeps, QPR and open the lid.

2. Set the IP to SAUTE. Cook till the mixture is simmering. Stir to mix. Shred the chicken right in the pot using 2 tongs; cook till the cooking liquid is reduced by 1/2. Stir in the remaining coconut cream; mix till smooth. Transfer to a serving dish; let cool for 5 up to 10 minutes before serving.

Seasoned Chicken

Servings|8   Prep. Time|**10 minutes**   Cook Time|**13 minutes**
Nutritional Content (per serving): Cal|**317**   Fat|**20.1g**   Protein|**31g**   Carbs|**2g**

1 teaspoon salt
1/2 cup water
1/4 cup olive oil
2 teaspoons garlic powder

2 teaspoons onion powder
3 teaspoons Italian seasoning
4 chicken breasts (boneless & skinless)

1. Put 1/2 of the olive oil in the IP. In a single layer, add the chicken to the pot. Drizzle the top with the remaining oil. Sprinkle the meat with 1/2 of the seasoning, flip, and sprinkle with the rest of the seasoning. Add the water. Lock the lid and close the pressure valve. Set to POULTRY for 13 minutes. When the timer beeps, QPR and open the lid.

2. Check the chicken if they are cooked through. Serve warm. You can dice or shred it. Use as needed; keep refrigerated or frozen.

PORK & LAMB

Pulled Pork BBQ

Servings|4 Prep. Time|10 minutes Cook Time|90-95 minutes
Nutritional Content (per serving): Cal|783 Fat|29.9g Protein|119.6g Carbs|3g

2.63 pounds pork roast
2 cups chicken stock or water
1/4 cup oil

Preferred lectin-free spices (pepper, salt, etc.)

1. Slice the pork into halves or size that is easy to handle and fir in your IP. Season the meat with preferred marinade, spices, or seasoning; let sit for 20 minutes.

2. Set the IP to SAUTÉ. Add the oil. When hot, add the pork; sear each side for 3 minutes. Add your preferred cooking liquid. Lock the lid and close the pressure valve. Set to MEAT/STEW for 90 minutes. When the timer beeps, press CANCEL, NPR for 10 minutes, then QPR and open the lid. Transfer the pork to a large plate or cutting board; shred using 2 forks. Serve.

Egg Roll Soup

Servings|4 Prep. Time|25 minutes Cook Time|25 minutes
Nutritional Content (per serving): Cal|334 Fat|8.7g Protein|41.4g Carbs|22.2g

1 onion, (large), diced
1 pound ground pork, pastured
1 tablespoon ghee, olive oil, or avocado oil
1 teaspoon garlic powder
1 teaspoon ginger (ground)
1 teaspoon onion powder

1 teaspoon sea salt
1/2 head cabbage, chopped
2 cups carrots, shredded
2/3 cup coconut aminos
2-3 tablespoons tapioca starch, optional
4 cups (32 ounces) chicken or beef broth

1. Set the IP to SAUTÉ. Add 1 tablespoon of cooking fat, the onion, and ground pork; cook till the meat is no longer pink. Add the rest of the ingredients. Lock the lid and close the pressure valve. Set to MANUAL HIGH for 25 minutes.

2. When the timer beeps, QPR and open the lid. To thicken the soup, scoop 1/4 cup of broth into a bowl (small). Whisk in the starch till smooth. Add the mixture to the pot; stir to mix well and till thickened.

Pork Roast w/ Apple Gravy

Servings|4   Prep. Time|**30 minutes**   Cook Time|**1 hour, 20 minutes**
Nutritional Content (per serving): Cal|**1233**   Fat|**85.8g**   Protein|**81.9g**   Carbs|**30.8g**

1 bay leaf
1 cup apple juice
1 cup chicken broth
1 piece (3 up to 5 pounds) pork shoulder roast (bone-in)
1 sprig rosemary (fresh)
1 tablespoon olive oil

1 teaspoon salt (kosher)
1 yellow onion, sliced
1/2 teaspoon pepper (fresh ground)
2 apples, core removed & sliced
3 sage (fresh) leaves
3 tablespoons butter
3 tablespoons cassava flour

1. Rinse the roast clean and dry thoroughly to help the meat crust nicely; season all the sides with pepper and salt. Set the IP to SAUTÉ. Add the oil. When hot, add the pork; cook each side for 5 minutes or till all sides are brown. Add the broth, apple juice, apples, bay leaf, rosemary, sage, and onion.

2. Lock the lid and close the pressure valve. Set the IP to MANUAL HIGH pressure for 60 minutes. When the timer beeps, press CANCEL, NPR completely, then QPR and open the lid.

3. Carefully transfer the pork to a plate; loosely tent with foil. Strain the solid out from the cooking juices through a fine mesh strainer; press the solids to squeeze out as much liquid as possible. Discard the solid; save the liquid for your gravy.

4. Return the inner pot to the housing – no need to clean and dry. Set the IP to SAUTÉ. Add the butter. When melted, add the flour; cook for 3 up to 5 minutes or till golden brown. Whisk in the cooking liquid; whisk till the texture is gravy-like. Shred the pork meat from the fat and bone; smother with the gravy.

Pork Shoulder

Servings|6   Prep. Time|**20 minutes**   Cook Time|**1 hour, 20 minutes**
Nutritional Content (per serving): Cal|**662**   Fat|**48.5g**   Protein|**52.8g**   Carbs|**0g**

3-5 pounds pork shoulder
2 cups cold water OR chicken or beef broth

Pork or ham base, optional
High smoking point lectin-free cooking oil

1. If your pork is frozen, thaw it overnight in your fridge before cooking time.

2. With the fat-side up, put the meat on a cutting board. Starting at one of the top edges, slice the pork shoulder where the thick fat layer is attached to the meat, adjusting your slicing point as needed. Once you find the right spot, hold your knife to around 45 to 90 degree angle with one hand. With your free hand, pull the fat back and slice off the cap, pulling the fat back as you

go. If preferred, you can leave the fat cap on and just remove it after cooking the meat. Slice the pork shoulder into 1 up to 2 pound chunks.

3. Set the IP to SAUTÉ. Add your preferred cooking oil. When hot, add the pork, cooking in batches so you do not overcrowd the pot and ensure there is a space between each piece. If you did not remove the fat cap, then put them in the pot with the fat cap-side down. Cook till every side of the meat is medium brown.

4. When you browned the last batch of meat, add the water; scrape the brown bits off the pot. Return the rest of the browned meat. Add the optional pork/ham base if using.

5. Lock the lid and close the pressure valve. Set to MANUAL HIGH pressure for 55 minutes. When the timer beeps, press CANCEL, NPR for 10 up to 15 minutes, then QPR and open the lid. Let the meat cool in the pot for 15 up to 20 minutes. Transfer to a plate using tongs. Let stand till cool enough to handle comfortably with your hands. If you did not remove the fat cap, then remove them. Shred the meat using your hands or 2 forks. Refrigerate or freeze leftover meat.

Ultimate Pot Roast

Servings|6   Prep. Time|**10 minutes**   Cook Time|**35 minutes**
Nutritional Content (per serving): Cal|**499**   Fat|**15.9g**   Protein|**49.8g**   Carbs|**30.4g**

1 cup red wine
1 cups beef broth
1 onion
2 stalks celery, chopped
2 tablespoons Italian Seasonings
2 tablespoons olive oil

2-3 pounds beef (chuck roast)
3 cloves garlic
4 carrots, chopped
4 sweet potatoes, (large), cut into large chunks

1. Set the IP to SAUTÉ. Add the oil and roast beef; cook the meat for 1 up to 2 minutes each side or till brown. Transfer the browned beef to a bowl. Put the potatoes, carrots, and celery in the pot. Put the beef on top the veggies. Sprinkle the seasoning on top of the meat.

2. Lock the lid and close the pressure valve. Set the IP to MANUAL HIGH pressure for 35 minutes. When the timer beeps, press CANCEL, NPR for 10-15 minutes, then QPR and open the lid. Serve.

Pork Sauerkraut

Servings|6 Prep. Time|**10 minutes** Cook Time|**30 minutes**
Nutritional Content (per serving): Cal|**403** Fat|**27.5g** Protein|**29g** Carbs|**9g**

24 ounces sauerkraut
14 ounces kielbasa, sliced
1/4 teaspoon pepper
1/3 cup water

1/2 teaspoon salt
1 tablespoon stevia
1 tablespoon oil
1 pounds country pork ribs

1. Set the IP to SAUTÉ. When hot, add the oil. Add all the pork ribs; season with pepper and salt. Cook till brown. Add the sauerkraut; sprinkle with the stevia. Put the kielbasa on top. Add the water – DO NOT STIR.

2. Lock the lid and close the pressure valve. Set to MANUAL HIGH pressure for 15 minutes. When the timer beeps, QPR or NPR and open the lid. Mix to combine the ingredients. Transfer to a serving dish; serve.

Pork Roast & Mushroom Gravy

Servings|8 Prep. Time|**20 minutes** Cook Time|**80-110 minutes**
Nutritional Content (per serving): Cal|**291** Fat|**14g** Protein|**34.3g** Carbs|**6.1g**

1 onion (medium), chopped
1 teaspoon sea or real salt
1/2teaspoon black pepper (fresh ground)
2 cups water
2 ribs celery

2 tablespoons coconut oil or ghee
2-3 pound (preferably a fatty) cut pork roast,
4 cloves garlic
4 cups cauliflower, chopped
8 ounces mushrooms (portabella), sliced

1. Put the cauliflower, onion, garlic, and celery in your IP. Add the water, Place the pork on top of the veggies season with pepper and salt. Lock the lid and close the pressure valve. Set to MANUAL HIGH pressure for 60 minutes for fully thawed or for 90 minutes frozen meat. When the timer beeps, QPR and open the lid.

2. Transfer the pork to an ovenproof dish. Bake in a preheated 400F oven till eh edges are crisped and the fat is rendered, making it similar to slow roasted pork. While the meat is roasting, transfer the cooking juices and all the veggies to your blender; puree till very smooth.

3. Set the IP to SAUTE – no need to wash the inner pot. Add the coconut oil and mushrooms; cook for 3 up to 5 minutes or till softened. Add the veggie puree; cook till desired thickness is achieved.

4. Remove the roasted pork from the oven. Shred the meat using 2 forks. Serve drizzled with the gravy.

Pulled Pork Tacos

Servings|8-10   Prep. Time|**10 minutes**   Cook Time|**60 minutes**
Nutritional Content (per serving): Cal|**681**   Fat|**48.9g**   Protein|**53.8g**   Carbs|**3.2g**

Pork:
1/2 teaspoon garlic powder
1/2 teaspoon cumin
1 yellow onion, (large), peeled & thinly sliced
1 teaspoon pepper (freshly ground)
1 piece (4 pounds) pork shoulder or butt, bone-in or bone-out)

1 cup chicken or beef broth
1 1/2 teaspoon sea salt
Lettuce leaves

Garnish:
Cilantro, chopped
Lime
Purple cabbage, sliced

1. Mix all of the spices in a bowl. Put the onion in your IP and add the broth. Rub all the sides of the pork with the spice blend. Add it to the pot. Lock the lid and close the pressure valve. Set tot MEAT for 60 minutes. When the timer beeps, QPR and open the lid.

2. Transfer the meat to a slicing board; discard the cooking juices and onion. Using 2 forks, shred the meat, discarding the fat in the process. If desired, you can broil the shredded pork in the oven for a few minutes or sear them in a hot pan to brown and crisp the edges. Top the meat in your lettuce leaves; garnish with purple cabbage and cilantro.

Pork Chops Topped w/ Apple Balsamic

Servings|**3**   Prep. Time|**5 minutes**   Cook Time|**35 minutes**
Nutritional Content (per serving): Cal|**400**   Fat|**18g**   Protein|**41g**   Carbs|**17g**

1 apple, cored & diced into chunks
1 tablespoon ghee
1 1/2 teaspoon garlic powder
1/2 onion, diced
1/2 teaspoon pepper

1/2 teaspoon salt
1/3 cup balsamic vinegar
3 thick cut (around 1-inch thick each) pork chops

1. Before you start cooking, prepare all the ingredients. Set the IP to SAUTE. Add the ghee. When melted, stir to coat the bottom. Add the pork; cook each side for 1 up to 2 minutes or till all sides are brown – just do a quick searing. Press CANCEL.

2. Sprinkle the apples and onion; drizzle with the vinegar. Season everything with the pepper, salt, and garlic powder. Lock the lid and close the pressure valve. Set to MANUAL for 10 minutes.

When the timer beeps, QPR and open the lid. Transfer the pork to a serving dish; spread the apple-onion mixture on top of each pork.

Kalua Pork w/ Bacon

Servings|8-10   Prep. Time|**10 minutes**   Cook Time|**1 hour, 30 minutes**
Nutritional Content (per serving): Cal|637   Fat|33g   Protein|78g   Carbs|3g

1 cup water
1 onion (large), roughly chopped
10 garlic cloves, peeled
5-pound pork roast (boneless), such as sirloin tip roast
6 slices bacon, cut into small pieces
Pepper & kosher salt

1. Set the IP to SAUTE. Add the bacon; cook till brown. Transfer to a plate. Do not drain the grease from the pot. Put the roast in the pot; cook till all the sides are brown. Transfer it to a dish; season with pepper and salt. Slice 10 slits in the sides of the meat and then tuck in 1 garlic clove inside each. Add the onion to the pot. Add the roast and water.

2. Lock the lid and close the pressure valve. Set to MANUAL HIGH pressure for 90 minutes. When the timer beeps, QPR and open the lid. Transfer the meat to a large plate or slicing board; shred using 2 forks. If desired, you can brown the meat in a pan/skillet till crisp.

Greek Ribs

Servings|6   Prep. Time|**2-4 hours, 20 minutes**   Cook Time|**65-70 minutes**
Nutritional Content (per serving): Cal|947   Fat|68g   Protein|82g   Carbs|3g

1 cup water, for cooking
1 tablespoon olive oil
1 tablespoon oregano (dried)
1 teaspoon pepper
2 racks (around 5 1/2 to 6 pounds) spare or baby back ribs
2 teaspoons salt
2 teaspoons smoked paprika
Juice of 2 lemons

1. Remove the membrane from the ribs; put them on a sheet pan lined with foil. In a bowl, mix the seasonings, lemon juice, and olive oil. Pour the mixture over the ribs; marinate in your fridge for 2 up to 4 hours.

2. Put the ribs and marinade in your IP. Add the water. Lock the lid and close the pressure valve. Set to MEAT/STEW HIGH pressure for 35 minutes. When the timer beeps, QPR and open the lid.

3. Carefully transfer to the prepared pan; pour some of the cooking juices over the ribs. Broil each side for 6 minutes on HIGH; watch carefully to avoid them from burning. Alternatively, you can grill the ribs and baste with the cooking sauce during cooking. Slice and serve.

Balsamic Rosemary Pork Tenderloin

Servings|4   Prep. Time|**7 minutes**   Cook Time|**47 minutes**
Nutritional Content (per serving): Cal|**270**   Fat|**8.25g**   Protein|**44.7g**   Carbs|**1.4g**

1 1/2 pounds quarter pork tenderloin
1 1/2 teaspoons balsamic vinegar
1 cup water, for the IP
1 teaspoon rosemary, dried

1 teaspoon salt (kosher)
1/4 teaspoons black pepper (fresh ground)
2 teaspoons olive oil
4 teaspoons minced garlic, cloves

1. Mix the garlic, pepper, salt, and rosemary in a bowl. Massage the pork with the seasonings. Whisk the olive oil and balsamic vinegar. Put the IP trivet and pour 1 cup water in the inner pot. Put the pork on the trivet. Pour the oil mixture on top of the meat. Lock the lid and close the pressure valve. Set to HIGH pressure for 20 minutes. When the timer beeps, press CANCEL, NPR completely, then QPR and open the lid. Serve.

Sausage & Kale

Servings|4   Prep. Time|**5 minutes**   Cook Time|**15 minutes**
Nutritional Content (per serving): Cal|**223**   Fat|**18g**   Protein|**12g**   Carbs|**0g**

1/4 cup water
4 smoked sausages
6 cups kale, collard greens, mustard greens, or preferred hearty greens, chopped

1. Put all of the ingredients in your IP. Lock the lid and close the pressure valve. Set to MANUAL HIGH pressure for 4 minutes. When the timer beeps, press CANCEL, NPR for 5 minutes, then QPR and open the lid.

4-Ingredient Sausage & Cabbage

Servings | **5**   Prep. Time | **10-15 minutes**   Cook Time | **20-25 minutes**
Nutritional Content (per serving): Cal | **623**   Fat | **42g**   Protein | **42g**   Carbs | **32g**

2 packages (19 ounces) sausage, sliced
1/2 cup broth or water
1 teaspoon minced garlic or 1 clove garlic
1 onion (small), sliced into small strips
1 head cabbage (small), cored & sliced into strips
Pepper & salt
1 tablespoon coconut oil

1. Set the IP to SAUTÉ. Add the oil, onion, and garlic; sauté till the onion is translucent. Add the cabbage. Add the sausage. Lock the lid and close the pressure valve. Set to MANUAL for 5 minutes. When the timer beeps, press CANCEL, NPR for 10 minutes, then QPR and open the lid. Serve.

Kalua Pork & Cabbage

Servings | **10**   Prep. Time | **10-15 minutes**   Cook Time | **120 minutes**
Nutritional Content (per serving): Cal | **487**   Fat | **23.1g**   Protein | **62g**   Carbs | **4.7g**

1 cup water
1 head cabbage, cored & sliced into 6 wedges
1 tablespoon salt (kosher)
3 slices bacon (thick-cut)
5 garlic cloves (whole), peeled
5-pound pork roast (shoulder/butt)

1. Cut the pork roast into 3 portions; score the fat cap side. With a pairing knife, cut 5 slits on the roast; stuff 1 garlic clove in each slit. Evenly sprinkle all the sides of the pork with salt.

2. Set the IP to SAUTÉ. Add the bacon; fry for 3 up to 5 minutes each side or till nicely brown. Set it in a single layer. Put the roast on top of the bacon. Add the water. Lock the lid and close the pressure valve. Set to HIGH pressure for 90 minutes.

3. When the timer beeps, press CANCEL, NPR completely, then QPR and open the lid. Transfer the roast to a bowl (large); shred using 2 forks. Add the solid contents of the pot to the bowl, leaving the cooking liquid; mix everything.

4. Put the cabbage in the IP. Lock the lid and close the pressure valve. Set to HIGH pressure for 5 minutes. When the timer beeps, QPR and open the lid. Add to the bowl with the pork mixture.

Lamb Leg

Servings|8-10   Prep. Time|5 minutes   Cook Time|35 minutes
Nutritional Content (per serving): Cal|264   Fat|12.6g   Protein|34.6g   Carbs|1.1g

1 boneless (3 to 4 pounds) lamb legs
2 cups water
2 tablespoon rosemary (fresh), chopped
2 tablespoons avocado oil, divided
4 cloves garlic, crushed
Pepper & salt

1. Pat dry the lamb with paper towels; season with pepper and salt. Set your IP to SAUTE. Add the oil. When hot, add the lamb and cook till all the sides brown. Transfer the lamb to a plate. Rub and spread the sides and top with the garlic and rosemary.

2. Put the IP trivet and pour the water into the inner pot. Put the lamb on the trivet. Lock the lid and close the pressure valve. Set to MEAT/STEW for 30 up to 35 minutes or depending on how done you want it. Thirty (30) minutes is enough to cook a 4-pound leg to medium-rare. When the timer beeps, press CANCEL, NPR completely, then QPR and open the lid.

3. Preheat your broiler. Put the lamb in a broiling pan; broil 6-inch from the heat source for 2 minutes or till the top is brown. Transfer to a serving dish; let rest for 10 minutes before slicing.

Lamb Shanks w/ Ginger & Figs

Servings|4   Prep. Time|20 minutes   Cook Time|90 minutes
Nutritional Content (per serving): Cal|560   Fat|20.1g   Protein|78.4g   Carbs|18g

1 1/2 cups bone broth
1 onion (large), sliced thinly from pole-to-pole
10 dried figs, stems sliced off & sliced lengthwise into halves
2 tablespoons coconut aminos
2 tablespoons coconut oil
2 tablespoons ginger (fresh), minced
2 tablespoons vinegar (apple cider)
2 teaspoons fish sauce
2-3 cloves garlic, finely minced
4 pieces (12-ounces each) lamb shanks

1. Set the IP to SAUTE. When hot, add 1 tablespoon of coconut oil. Put 2 lamb shanks in the pot; cook till all the sides are brown, occasionally turning. Transfer to a bowl or plate. Repeat the process with the remaining coconut oil and lamb shanks.

2. Put the ginger and onion to the empty IP; cook for 3 minutes or till soft, stirring often. Stir in the vinegar, fish, sauce, coconut aminos, and garlic. Pour in the broth and add the figs; scrape the browned bits off the pot. Add the shanks and any accumulated meat juices, making sure that the meaty portion of each shank is at least partially submerged in the cooking liquid. Lock the lid and close the pressure valve. Set to HIGH pressure for 1 hour. When the timer beeps, press CANCEL, NPR for 20 up to 30 minutes, then QPR and open the lid.

3. Transfer the shanks to a serving dish. Skim the fat off the surface of the cooking liquid and discard. Ladle the defatted sauce over the shanks. Serve over cauliflower rice.

BEEF

Beef & Broccoli

Servings|4   Prep. Time|20 minutes   Cook Time|30 minutes
Nutritional Content (per serving): Cal|267   Fat|7.5g   Protein|37.9g   Carbs|9.3g

1 clove garlic, (large), crushed/pressed
1 onion, quartered
1 pound stewing beef meat
1 teaspoon ginger (ground)
1/2 cup beef/bone broth

1/2 teaspoon salt
1/4 cup coconut aminos
10-12 ounces frozen broccoli (bagged)
2 tablespoons fish sauce

1. Except for your broccoli, put the rest of your ingredients in the IP. Lock the lid and close the pressure valve. Set the MEAT/STEW and cook on preset cooking time. When the timer beeps, QPR and open the lid. Add the broccoli. Loosely cover the IP with the lid; let sit for 15 minutes or till the broccoli is cooked to the desired doneness with the residual heat. Serve.

Beef Short Ribs

Servings|6   Prep. Time|25 minutes   Cook Time|35 minutes
Nutritional Content (per serving): Cal|705   Fat|32.3g   Protein|89.4g   Carbs|8.6g

1 1/2 cups beef broth
1 tablespoon thyme (dried)
2 cups onions, diced
2 tablespoons olive oil

3 cloves garlic, minced
4 pounds beef short ribs
4-6 carrots, cut into bite-sized chunks
Salt (kosher) & pepper (fresh cracked)

1. Set the IP to SAUTÉ. Pat dry the beef meat; generously season them with salt and pepper. Add the oil to the pot. In batches of a single layer at a time, cook the beef in the pot for 4 up to 5 minutes per side or till every side are brown. Transfer the browned beef to a plate; set aside.

2. Put the garlic in the pot; stir for 1 minute. Add the carrot, onion, and thyme, season with more pepper and salt as needed. Cook for 4 up to 5 minutes or till the veggies are soft, occasionally stirring. Return the browned beef in the pot.

3. Lock the lid and close the pressure valve. Set the MANUAL HIGH pressure for 35 minutes. When the timer beeps, press CANCEL, NPR for 10 up to 15 minutes, then QPR and open the lid. Serve hot.

Braised Beef Short Ribs

Servings|8   Prep. Time|30 minutes   Cook Time|35 minutes
Nutritional Content (per serving): Cal|482   Fat|21.2g   Protein|66.4g   Carbs|1.7g

4 pounds beef short ribs, or more as desired
3 cloves garlic
1 tablespoon bacon or beef fat, or avocado oil or preferred vegetable oil
1 onion, skin on, quartered
Salt (kosher)
Water

1. Generously season all the sides with the salt. Set the IP to SAUTÉ. Add the oil. When hot, add a few pieces of ribs at a time in the pot so you do not overcrowd it; cook till all the sides are evenly and nicely brown. Transfer the browned ribs to a plate as you cook. When the last batch of ribs is brown, return the rest in the pot, along with any accumulated meat juices.

2. Add 2-inch worth of water in the IP. Add the onion and garlic. Lock the lid and close the pressure valve. Set to MANUAL HIGH pressure for 35 minutes. When the timer beeps, QPR and open the lid. Transfer the ribs to a serving dish using tongs. Serve the ribs on bone or pull the meat off the bones; save the bones for broth. Strain the cooking juices, and skim off the fat. Season the broth to taste. Serve with the ribs.

Braised Beef Ribs

Servings|4-6   Prep. Time|5 minutes   Cook Time|75 minutes
Nutritional Content (per serving): Cal|993   Fat|31.9g   Protein|141g   Carbs|25.1g

1 tablespoon sesame oil
1/3 cup stevia
1/4 cup vinegar (white balsamic)
1-2 tablespoons water
1-inch knob ginger (fresh), peeled & finely chopped
2 cloves garlic, peeled & crushed/smashed
2 tablespoons tapioca starch
2/3 cup salt-free beef stock (homemade)
2/3 cup soy sauce tamari/coconut aminos
4 pounds beef ribs (around 8 pieces), ask your butcher to chop or saw them into halves

1. Set the IP to SAUTÉ. Add the oil. When hot, add the ginger and garlic; sauté for 1 minute. Add the stock, stevia, coconut aminos, and vinegar; stir to mix well. Add the ribs; stir to coat with the stock mixture. Lock the lid and close the pressure valve. Set the IP to MANUAL HIGH pressure for 45 up to 60 minutes.

2. When the timer beeps, press CANCEL, NPR for 10 up to 15 minutes, then QPR and open the lid. Transfer the ribs to a baking sheet; broil for 5 minutes or till rich dark brown. Meanwhile, mix the water and starch till smooth. Set the IP to SAUTÉ. Add the slurry to the cooking juices

and boil; cook till desired texture is achieved. Pour over the broiled ribs. Serve with steamed broccoli.

Smoked Maple Brisket

Servings|**2**   Prep. Time|**30 minutes**   Cook Time|**50 minutes**
Nutritional Content (per serving): Cal|**750**   Fat|**23.5g**   Protein|**109.1g**   Carbs|**19.4g**

3 thyme sprigs (fresh)
2 cups bone broth or preferred stock
1 tablespoon liquid smoke
1 1/2 pounds beef brisket

Spice mix:
1 teaspoon black pepper (fresh ground)
1 teaspoon onion powder
1/2 teaspoon paprika (smoked)
2 tablespoons coconut sugar or stevia
1 teaspoon mustard powder
2 teaspoons salt (smoked sea)

1. Thirty (30) minutes just before cooking time, remove your beef from the fridge. Pat dry the meat using paper towels. In a bowl, mix all the spice mix ingredients. Generously season all the sides of the meat with the blend.

2. Set the IP to SAUTÉ; let heat for 2 up to 3 minutes. Add high heat lectin-free cooking oil to coat the bottom of the pot. Add the brisket; cook till all the sides are deep golden, and not burnt. When all the sides of the meat are browned, turn it so the fatty side is up. Add your liquid smoke, broth, and thyme. Scrape off the browned morsels from the pot.

3. Lock the lid and close the pressure valve. Set to MANUAL HIGH pressure for 50 minutes. When the timer beeps, press CANCEL, NPR completely, then QPR and open the lid. Transfer the beef to a serving dish; cover with foil and let rest.

4. Set the IP to SAUTÉ; cook the cooking liquid for 10 minutes or till thick and reduced. Slice the meat diagonally across the grain. Serve with a favorite mashed veggie and then drizzle with sauce.

Beef Back Ribs

Servings|**2**   Prep. Time|**5 minutes**   Cook Time|**30 minutes**
Nutritional Content (per serving): Cal|**1806**   Fat|**97g**   Protein|**211g**   Carbs|**7.5g**

4 ounces applesauce (unsweetened)
3/4 cup water
2 tablespoons coconut aminos
1 teaspoon fish sauce

1 rack (around 3.5 pounds) beef back ribs
Preferred dry rub
Salt (kosher

1. Pat dry the ribs. Liberally season both sides with the dry rub and then the salt. Wrap them with foil and refrigerate for at least 2 hours up to 24 hours to marinate.

2. Place an oven rack about 4 to 6-inch from the heat source; preheat your broiler. Slice the racks into 3 even portions. Put the ribs on a wire rack set on a sheet pan lined with foil. Broil them for 1 up to 2 minutes per side or till nicely charred. Remove the ribs from the broiler; keep the broiler on to cook the ribs at the end.

3. Put the water, applesauce, coconut aminos, and fish sauce in the IP; stir to mix. Set a clean trivet in the pot. Pile the ribs on the trivet. Lock the lid and close the pressure valve. Set to MANUAL HIGH pressure for 20 minutes. When the timer beeps, QPR and open the lid.

4. Transfer the ribs to a wire rack set on a sheet pan lined with foil.

5. Set the IP to SAUTÉ. Simmer the cooking liquid for 5 minutes or till reduced to 2 cups. Skim the fat off the surface if desired. Adjust the seasoning as needed. Press CANCEL and unplug your IP. Baste the beef ribs with the sauce; broil for 1 minute or till crunchy.

Corned Beef w/ Cabbage & Carrots

Servings|12   Prep. Time|15 minutes   Cook Time|1 hour, 15 minutes
Nutritional Content (per serving): Cal|317   Fat|9.7g   Protein|47.3g   Carbs|8.1g

1 cup (around 2 pieces) 2 onions, sliced
1 cup (around 4 pieces) carrots, sliced into thirds
1 cup (around 4 stalks) celery, chopped
1 head cabbage, cut into wedges (8 cups)
2 teaspoons black peppercorns (fresh ground)
2 teaspoons mustard (dried)
4 cloves garlic
4 pounds corned beef brisket
6 cups water

1. Put the beef in your IP; discard the spice packet that is packed with the meat. Add the water to the pot; adding more as needed to cover the beef. Add the spices. Lock the lid and close the pressure valve. Set to MEAT/STEW HIGH pressure for 60 minutes. When the timer beeps, press CANCEL, NPR completely, then QPR and open the lid. Transfer the beef to a serving dish; cover with foil to keep warm.

2. Add the veggies to the IP. Lock the lid and close the pressure valve. Set to SOUP for 15 minutes. When the timer beeps, QPR and open the lid. Return the beef to the pot; let warm. Serve.

3-Ingredient Pot Roast

Servings|**10-12**   Prep. Time|**15 minutes**   Cook Time|**110 minutes**
Nutritional Content (per serving): Cal|**359**   Fat|**18g**   Protein|**48.4g**   Carbs|**0.45g**

1/2 cup water
2 tablespoons avocado oil, ghee, or preferred lectin-free cooking fat
2 teaspoons garlic powder
2 teaspoons salt (fine sea)
4 up to 5-pound beef roast
Black pepper (fresh ground), to taste

1. Set the IP to SAUTE. Let heat for 2 minutes. Season 1 side of the roast with 1/2 of the black pepper, garlic powder, and salt. Add the cooking fat to the pot. Carefully put the roast in the pot with the seasoned-side down. Cook for 10 minutes. Season the top side of the meat with the remaining salt, pepper, and garlic powder. Flip the meat. Press CANCEL.

2. Add the water to the pot. Lock the lid and close the pressure valve. Set to MEAT/STEW for 85 minutes. When the timer beeps, press CANCEL, NPR completely, then QPR and open the lid. Transfer the roast to a serving dish; leave the cooking liquid in the pot. Serve the meat.

Corned Beef w/ Cabbage & Carrots

Servings|**6**   Prep. Time|**5 minutes**   Cook Time|**2 hours**
Nutritional Content (per serving): Cal|**447**   Fat|**28.5g**   Protein|**32.7g**   Carbs|**14.5g**

5 carrots, (medium), peeled & sliced into chunks
4 cups water
3 whole black peppercorns (fresh ground)
3 garlic cloves, peeled & smashed
2 bay leaves
1/2 teaspoon allspice berries (whole)
1 teaspoon thyme (dried)
1 piece (3-4 pounds) corned beef brisket
1 onion, (small), peeled & quartered
1 head cabbage, sliced into wedges

1. Put the beef, onion, peppercorns, garlic, thyme, and allspice in your IP. Lock the lid and close the pressure valve. Set to MANUAL HIGH pressure for 90 minutes. When the timer beeps, press CANCEL, NPR for 10 minutes, then QPR and open the lid. Transfer the beef to a serving dish; cover with foil and let rest for 15 minutes.

2. Meanwhile, add the carrots and cabbage in the IP. Lock the lid and close the pressure valve. Set to MANUAL HIGH pressure for 10 minutes. When the timer beeps, QPR and open the lid. Transfer the cooked veggies to the serving dish with beef using a slotted spoon. Moisten the meat and veggies with some of the cooking juices as needed. Serve.

Pot Roast

Servings | **4-8**   Prep. Time | **30 minutes**   Cook Time | **90 minutes**
Nutritional Content (per serving): Cal | **719**   Fat | **19.9g**   Protein | **83.8g**   Carbs | **45.3g**

8 ounces white mushrooms, sliced into halves
2-3 pounds boneless (or 3-4 pounds bone-in) chuck roast
2 tablespoons ghee
1/4 teaspoon black pepper (fresh ground)
1/4 cup red wine or 1 tablespoons red wine vinegar
1/2 teaspoon salt (kosher)
1 yellow onion (small), chopped
1 tablespoons fish sauce
1 pound carrots, sliced into bite-sized chunks
1 cup chicken broth
1 cup beef broth
1 clove garlic, minced
1 1/2 pounds sweet potatoes, sliced into bite-sized chunks
Pepper & salt, to taste

1. Generously season the roast with pepper and salt. Put the ghee in your IP. Set to SAUTE. When hot, add the roast; cook for 6 minutes or till the underside is brown and easily pulls away from the pot. Flip and cook for 6 minutes till the other side is brown. Transfer the roast to a dish; set aside.

2. Put the onion in the IP; sauté for 4 minutes or till soft, stirring often. Add the garlic; stir for 30 seconds or till aromatic. Add the beef and chicken broth, and wine. Stir to mix and simmer. Once simmering, add the roast and any accumulated meat juices. Lock the lid and close the pressure valve. Set to STEW/MEAT HIGH pressure for 45 minutes. When the timer beeps, press CANCEL, NPR for 10 minutes, then QPR and open the lid. Transfer the meat to a rimmed sheet pan; set aside.

3. Put the mushrooms, potatoes, and carrots in the IP. Lock the lid and close the pressure valve. Set to STEW/MEAT HIGH pressure for 6 minutes. While the veggies are cooking, roast the meat in your oven for 4 minutes or till the top is crisped and fat is rendered. Transfer to a clean slicing board; loosely tent with foil to keep warm.

4. When the timer beeps, QPR and open the lid. Transfer the veggies to a sheet pan using a slotted spoon. Set the IP to SAUTE. Bring the contents of the pot to a simmer. Cook till the cooking juices is reduced.

5. Meanwhile, broil the veggies in your oven for 5 minutes, flipping and jostling the pan every few minutes. Slice the roast and transfer to a serving dish. Add the roasted veggies to the dish as well. When the cooking juices is reduced, season as needed with pepper and salt. Pour some of the sauce over the veggies and meat. Serve with the rest of the sauce as gravy.

Mongolian Beef with Carrots

Servings|4   Prep. Time|15 minutes   Cook Time|35 minutes
Nutritional Content (per serving): Cal|338   Fat|15g   Protein|37g   Carbs|11g

1 1/2 pounds flank steak, sliced
1/2 cups carrot, grated
1/2 teaspoons ginger (fresh), peeled & minced
1/3 cup scallion (green onion), diced

1/4 cups arrowroot flour
2 tablespoons olive oil
3/4 cups coconut aminos
3/4 cups stevia
3/4 cups water

1. Coat the meat with the flour. Mix the green onion, carrots, honey, water, coconut aminos, ginger, and olive oil in your IP. Put the steak in the pot. Lock the lid and close the pressure valve. Set to HIGH pressure for 35 minutes. When the timer beeps, press CANCEL, NPR for 5 minutes, then QPR and open the lid. Serve.

Mongolian Beef

Servings|4   Prep. Time|3 minutes   Cook Time|17 minutes
Nutritional Content (per serving): Cal|486   Fat|17.7g   Protein|50.6g   Carbs|29.1g

3/4 cup coconut aminos/tamari
1/4 cup water
1/2 teaspoon ginger (fresh), minced
1/2 cup stevia
1 tablespoon olive oil
1 green onion, sliced, for garnish
1 garlic clove, minced

1 carrot, shredded
1 1/2 pounds flank steak

To thicken:
3 tablespoons tapioca starch
3 tablespoons water

1. Slice the flank into thin strips. In a bowl, mix the water, sugar, ginger, garlic, oil; pour the sauce in the IP. Add the beef strips and carrot; mix till well coated with the sauce. Lock the lid and close the pressure valve. Set to MANUAL HIGH pressure for 8 minutes.

2. When the timer beeps, press CANCEL, NPR completely, then QPR and open the lid. In a bowl (small). Mix the starch and water till smooth. Set the IP to SAUTÉ. Pour the mixture into the pot; boil for 1 up to 2 minutes or till the sauce is thick. Transfer to a serving dish; garnish with green onions.

Beef Chili

Servings|4-6   Prep. Time|**20 minutes**   Cook Time|**60 minutes**
Nutritional Content (per serving): Cal|**510**   Fat|**18g**   Protein|**39g**   Carbs|**48g**

1 large (around 2 1/2 cups) beet, peeled & chopped fined
1 onion (medium), diced
1 pound ground beef (grass-fed)
1 sweet potato (medium/large), peeled and chopped, around 2 cups
1 teaspoon oregano (dried)
1/2 avocado, sliced, for garnish, optional
1/2 teaspoon sea salt
2 teaspoons cilantro (fresh), for garnish, optional
3 cloves garlic, minced
3 medium carrots, peeled & chopped
4 cups bone broth

1. Set the IP to SAUTE. Add the beef; cook till brown. Add the rest of the ingredients, reserving the avocado and cilantro for garnish; stir to mix the contents of the pot. Lock the lid and close the pressure valve. Set to MANUAL for 35 minutes. When the timer beeps, QPR and open the lid. Serve. Garnish with avocado and cilantro.

Very Simple 5-Ingredient Corned Beef

Servings|6   Prep. Time|**5 minutes**   Cook Time|**90 minutes**
Nutritional Content (per serving): Cal|**461**   Fat|**34g**   Protein|**34g**   Carbs|**3g**

1 onion, quartered
2 bay leaves
3 cloves garlic, peeled
3 pounds corned beef brisket
Water or dill pickle juice

1. Rinse the beef brisket. Put it in your IP along with its spice packet, onion, garlic, and bay leaves. Add enough water to cover the meat. Lock the lid and close the pressure valve. Set to MANUAL HIGH pressure for 90 minutes. When the timer beeps, press CANCEL, NPR for 10 5 minutes, then QPR and open the lid.

2. Transfer the beef to a serving dish, leaving the other items in the pot. If you want to cook veggies, then save the cooking liquid in the IP. Add your cabbage, carrots and sweet potatoes. Lock the lid and close the pressure valve. Set to MANUAL HIGH pressure for 5 minutes.

3. Shred the meat. Serve with the cooked veggies.

Beef & Broccoli w/ Carrots

Servings|4-6   Prep. Time|15 minutes   Cook Time|15 minutes
Nutritional Content (per serving): Cal|201   Fat|8.4g   Protein|17.3g   Carbs|15g

1 cup carrots, shredded
1 flank (around 1 1/2 - 2 pounds) steak, sliced against the grain into thin, long strips
1 onion (small), diced
1 tablespoon avocado oil, divided
1 teaspoon sesame oil
1/2 cup coconut aminos
1/2 cup water
2 tablespoons coconut sugar or stevia

2 tablespoons tapioca starch dissolved in 2 tablespoons cold water
3 garlic cloves
6-8 cups broccoli
Juice of 1 lime
Pepper & salt to taste

Toppings:
Green onions
Sesame seeds

1. Set the IP to SAUTE LESS mode. When hot, add 1/2 tablespoon avocado oil. When hot, add the broccoli; stir to coat with oil. Saute for 5 minutes or till they start to soften and turn bright green. Transfer to a bowl; set aside.

2. Set the IP to SAUTE MORE mode. Add the remaining 1/2 tablespoon avocado oil. When hot, add the onion; saute till soft. Add the meat; cook for 2 up to 3 minutes or till brown. Add the water, coconut aminos, coconut sugar/stevia, and garlic; stir to mix. Add the carrots on top of the meat.

3. Lock the lid and close the pressure valve. Set to MANUAL HIGH pressure for 10 minutes. When the timer beeps, QPR and open the lid. Keep the IP on KEEP WARM mode. Mix the starch with the water till smooth. Add the mixture to the pot. Add the lime juice, sesame oil, and broccoli; season with pepper and salt as needed. Stir to mix; let sit for 5 minutes or till the sauce is thick. Serve over cauliflower rice; garnish with sesame seeds and green onions.

Delicious Crispy Beef Tongue

Servings|5   Prep. Time|15 minutes   Cook Time|45 minutes, plus frying
Nutritional Content (per serving): Cal|675   Fat|50g   Protein|41g   Carbs|11g

1 beef tongue (whole)
1 teaspoon cumin, optional
1 teaspoon garlic powder, optional
2-3 tablespoons coconut oil

2-3 teaspoons sea salt
3 cups water
Black pepper (fresh ground), to taste

1. Put the beef tongue and water in the IP. Lock the lid and close the pressure valve. Set to STEW for 35 minutes. When the timer beeps, press CANCEL, NPR for 30 minutes, then QPR and open

the lid. Transfer the tongs to a cutting board using tongs. When cool enough to handle, peel the tongue, making a slice through the skin to start.

2. Starting at the tip, slice the tongue at an angle into 1/2-inch slices. Heat a pan/skillet over medium-high flame/heat. Add 1 tablespoon of coconut oil; spread it around. Put the slices of tongue close together in the pan; season with 1 teaspoon salt and optional pepper to taste if using. Cook for 5 minutes. Lower the flame/heat to medium; cook for 3 minutes or till the underside is crisp. Flip, lightly season the top side with salt and pepper. Fry till the other side is crisp. Transfer to a plate. Repeat the process with any remaining meat.

3. Transfer the cooked tongue to a slicing board; cut them into strips as desired. Serve as desired.

4-Ingredient Corned Beef w/ Cabbage & Carrots

Servings|4   Prep. Time|**5 minutes**   Cook Time|**1 hour, 35 minutes**
Nutritional Content (per serving): Cal|**820**   Fat|**60g**   Protein|**60g**   Carbs|**9g**

1 head (small) green cabbage, cut into 8 wedges
2 cups baby carrots

3 1/2 pounds corned beef brisket (including spices)
5 cups water

1. If your corned beef is uncured, leave it as is. If it is cured, then drain and rinse. Put the beef in your IP, along with the spices. Add around 5 cups of water or just enough to level with the top of the meat. Push on the meat with your hands to flatten it as needed. Lock the lid and close the pressure valve. Set to MANUAL HIGH pressure for 90 minutes. When the timer beeps, QPR and open the lid.

2. The beef is cooked through if a fork easily pierces through the thickest part of the meat. If not, pressure cook on HIGH for 10 minutes. Test again. Without removing the meat, add the carrots and cabbage – do not overfill the pot beyond its maximum capacity. Lock the lid and close the pressure valve. Set to MANUAL HIGH pressure for 5 minutes.

3. When the timer beeps, QPR and open the lid. Transfer the beef to a serving platter; slice against the grain into thick slices. Transfer the veggies to a serving platter. Serve.

Beef & Broccoli

Servings|**4**   Prep. Time|**20 minutes**   Cook Time|**30 minutes**
Nutritional Content (per serving): Cal|**179**   Fat|**5.17g**   Protein|**29g**   Carbs|**6g**

1 large clove garlic, pressed
1 onion, quartered
1 pound beef stew meat (grass fed)
1 teaspoon ginger (ground)
1/2 cup beef or bone broth

1/2 teaspoon salt
1/4 cup coconut aminos
10 to 12 ounces organic broccoli (bagged, frozen)
2 tablespoons fish sauce

1. Except for the broccoli, put the rest of the ingredients in the IP. Lock the lid and close the pressure valve. Set to MEAT/STEW and cook on preset cooking time. When the timer beeps, QPR and open the lid. Press CANCEL. Add the broccoli. Cover with the lid. Let sit for 15 minutes to cook the broccoli with the residual heat. Uncover. Stir to mix. Serve.

Balsamic Roast Beef

Servings|**5-10**   Prep. Time|**5-10 minutes**   Cook Time|**1 hour**
Nutritional Content (per serving): Cal|**321**   Fat|**11g**   Protein|**44g**   Carbs|**9g**

1 1/2 teaspoon truffle salt or salt
1 cup beef broth
1 tablespoon coconut aminos
1 tablespoon fish sauce
1 tablespoon honey
1 tablespoon olive oil (extra-virgin)

1/2 cup balsamic vinegar
1/2 teaspoon rosemary and/or lavender (dried), optional
3-4 pounds shoulder or chuck roast
4 cloves garlic, crushed

1. Pat dry the roast using paper towels; rub all the sides of the pork with the salt. Put the olive oil in the IP. Set the IP to SAUTE. Add the roast; sear each side for 2-3 minutes or till brown. Add the rest of the ingredients in the pot. Lock the lid and close the pressure valve. Set to HIGH pressure for 45 minutes. Transfer the roast to a serving dish; tent with foil and let rest for 5 up to 10 minutes.

2. Meanwhile, set the IP to SAUTE. Cook the juices in the pot for about 10 minutes or till reduced to about 2/3; keep an eye on it. Slice the roast and drizzle the sauce over it. Garnish with salt and parsley.

Italian Beef

Servings|6   Prep. Time|**5 minutes**   Cook Time|**2 hours, 5 minutes**
Nutritional Content (per serving): Cal|**279**   Fat|**9g**   Protein|**44g**   Carbs|**4g**

1 cup beef broth
1 teaspoon basil
1 teaspoon marjoram
1 teaspoon onion powder
1 teaspoon oregano
1 teaspoon salt (Himalayan pink)

1/2 teaspoon ginger (ground)
1/4 cup vinegar (apple cider)
2 teaspoons garlic powder
3 pounds chuck roast (grass-fed)
6 cloves garlic

1. With a sharp knife, preferably pairing, cut 6 slits in the meat; stuff each with 1 garlic cloves. Whisk the salt, marjoram, basil, oregano, ginger, onion powder, and garlic powder till well mixed. Rub all the sides of the roast with the spice rub. Put in the IP.

2. Add the broth and the vinegar. Lock the lid and close the pressure valve. Set to MANUAL to 90 minutes. When the timer beeps, press CANCEL, NPR for 20 minutes, then QPR and open the lid. Transfer the beef to a large plate or cutting board; shred using caveman claws or 2 forks. Moisten with some of the cooking juice if desired.

Beef Brisket

Servings|4   Prep. Time|**45 minutes**   Cook Time|**1 hour**
Nutritional Content (per serving): Cal|**403**   Fat|**16g**   Protein|**47g**   Carbs|**7g**

2 pounds beef brisket
2 cloves garlic, peeled & halved
1/4 cup beef or chicken stock
1/2 teaspoon thyme (dried)
1/2 teaspoon oregano (dried)
1 teaspoon onion powder

1 teaspoon garlic powder
1 teaspoon coarse sea salt, or to taste
1 tablespoon stevia
1 tablespoon bacon fat or preferred cooking fat
1 onion, peeled & sliced

1. Set your IP to SAUTÉ. Add the bacon fat, onion, and garlic; sauté till the onion is translucent. Stir in the thyme, oregano, onion powder, garlic powder, and salt; cook for 2 minutes. Transfer to a bowl (small); set aside.

2. Mix the stock and stevia in your IP; scrape the browned bits off the pot. Add the beef; spread the onion mixture on top of the meat. Lock the lid and close the pressure valve. Set to HIGH pressure for 50 minutes. When the timer beeps, press CANCEL, NPR completely or QPR and open the lid.

3. While the beef is still hot, scrape off any fat on the meat using a spoon and discard. Transfer the meat, along with all the cooking juices to a baking dish. Refrigerate the brisket for a couple of hours up to 1 day; this process with enhance the texture and flavor of the beef significantly. After resting the meat, remove from the fridge. Remove as much solidified fat from the meat as desired.

4. Transfer the beef to a slicing board; sliced against in grain into 1/2-inch slices. Puree the cooking juices using a stick blender of s stand blender till smooth. Put the meat and the sauce back in your IP. Lock the lid and close the pressure valve. Set to HIGH pressure for 3 minutes to warm. When the timer beeps, press CANCEL, NPR completely or QPR and open the lid. Serve with lectin-free fresh salad.

2-Ingredient Ground Beef

Servings | **4-8**   Prep. Time | **5 minutes**   Cook Time | **15-22 minutes**
Nutritional Content (per serving): Cal | **495**   Fat | **26g**   Protein | **62g**   Carbs | **0g**

2-4 pounds ground beef (frozen or fresh)   1 cup beef broth

1. Put the ground beef in the IP. Add the broth. Lock the lid and close the pressure valve. Set to HIGH pressure for 22 minutes for frozen or for 15 minutes for fresh. When the timer beeps, press CANCEL, NPR for 10 minutes, then QPR and open the lid. Break the meat using a wooden spoon and drain off the cooking liquid; store properly till using.

Beef Barbacoa

Servings | **6-8**   Prep. Time | **5 minutes**   Cook Time | **1 hour, 5 minutes**
Nutritional Content (per serving): Cal | **358**   Fat | **14g**   Protein | **52g**   Carbs | **4g**

1 cup beef or bone broth
1 onion (large), quartered
1 tablespoon cumin
1 tablespoon oregano (dried)
1/2 teaspoon black pepper (ground)
1/4 cup lime juice
1/4 cup vinegar (apple cider, raw & unfiltered)

2 tablespoons coconut oil
2 teaspoons sea salt
3-4 pounds (chuck or round roast) beef bottom, chopped into 3-inch chunks
5 garlic cloves
Cilantro (fresh), for garnish

1. Set your IP to SAUTÉ. Add the coconut oil; heat for 10 minutes. Add the beef; cook each side for 5 minutes or till all side till brown, working in batches as needed. When all the beef is browned, put them all in the pot and turn off your IP.

2. Except for the cilantro, blend the rest of the ingredients in your blender till smooth. Pour the sauce over the meat. Lock the lid and close the pressure valve. Set to HIGH pressure for 60 minutes. When the timer beeps, press CANCEL, NPR for 10 up to 15 minutes, then QPR and open the lid.

3. Transfer the beef to a large plate or cutting board; shred the meat using 2 forks and return to the pot. Stir to mix with the cooking juices. Sprinkle with cilantro. Serve in your burrito bowl, as taco meat, or in any dish.

STOCKS & SAUCES

Chicken Stock

Servings | **4 liters**   Prep. Time | **5 minutes**   Cook Time | **120 minutes**
Nutritional Content (per serving): Cal | **162**   Fat | **5.8g**   Protein | **20.5g**   Carbs | **3.9g**

2 tablespoons vinegar (apple cider)
2 bay leaves
10-15 pieces whole peppercorns
1 onion, sliced into quarters
1 chicken carcass

Veggie scraps, optional
Water

Equipment:
4-5 mason jars

1. Put the chicken carcass in your IP. Add some skin if preferred. Add the rest of the ingredients. Add enough water to fill your IP 1/2-inch below the max line. Lock the lid and close the pressure valve. Set to SOUP for 120 minutes.

2. When the timer beeps, press CANCEL, NPR for 10 up to 15 minutes; let sit for at least 30 minutes without releasing the pressure. QPR and open the lid. Strain the stock; discarding all the debris. Transfer the stock to the mason jars without overfilling them. Let cool. Refrigerate if using within 3 days. Freeze if storing for long periods. If freezing, use 5 mason jars.

Beef & Chicken Bone Broth

Servings | **4 liters**   Prep. Time | **5 minutes**   Cook Time | **120 minutes**
Nutritional Content (per serving): Cal | **162**   Fat | **5.8g**   Protein | **20.5g**   Carbs | **3.9g**

1 tablespoons vinegar (apple cider)
Bay leaf
Beef and chicken bones, enough to fill the pot

Filtered water
Handful peppercorns
Onions, celery, & carrots

1. Put the beef bones in your IP. Put the chicken bones on top. Add the rest of the ingredients. Fill the pot with water – do not fill more than 2/3 full. Lock the lid and close the pressure valve. Set to MANUAL HIGH pressure for 120 minutes. When the timer beeps, press CANCEL, NPR completely, then QPR and open the lid. Strain the broth and store in jars.

Fish & Vegetable Stock

Servings|**3 quarts**   Prep. Time|**20 minutes**   Cook Time|**45 minutes**
Nutritional Content (per serving): Cal|**42**   Fat|**2g**   Protein|**5.6g**   Carbs|**0g**

1 cup carrots, roughly chopped
1 cup celery, roughly chopped
2 cloves garlic
2 lemongrass stalks, roughly chopped

2 salmon heads (large), sliced into quarters
Handful thyme (fresh), including stems
Oil, for frying

1. Wash the fish heads under cold running water, making sure there is no blood. Pat them dry after washing. Put the oil in your IP. Set to SAUTÉ. Add the fish heads and lightly sear – this will minimize them from falling apart. Transfer the fish head to a bowl. Spread the veggies on the bottom of the IP. Place the fish heads and thyme on top. Add 3 quarts of water or just enough to cover the fish.

2. Lock the lid and close the pressure valve. Set to SOUP HIGH pressure for 45 minutes. When the timer beeps, press CANCEL, NPR for 10 up to 15 minutes, then QPR and open the lid. Strain the stock and store properly.

Beef Bone Broth

Servings|**8**   Prep. Time|**5 minutes**   Cook Time|**90 minutes**
Nutritional Content (per serving): Cal|**18**   Fat|**0.6g**   Protein|**2.9g**   Carbs|**0.1g**

1 onion, roughly chopped
3 bay leaves
3 pounds beef bones (neck bones or oxtail preferred)
4 cloves garlic

4-5 sprigs thyme
5 ounces carrots
Half head celery, chopped
Pepper to taste
Salt to taste

1. Slice the onion and celery. Add them to your IP. Add the rest of the ingredients. Fill the pot with water up to the max line. Lock the lid and close the pressure valve. Set to MANUAL HIGH pressure for 90 minutes. When the timer beeps, QPR and open the lid. Strain the broth and store properly.

Pork & Chicken Bone Broth

Servings|**8 cups**   Prep. Time|**20 minutes**   Cook Time|**30-50 minutes**
Nutritional Content (per serving): Cal|**13**   Fat|**0.3g**   Protein|**2g**   Carbs|**0.9g**

8 cups water (enough to fill the IP 2/3rd its capacity)
2 tablespoons fish
2 leeks (medium), cleaned & sliced crosswise into halves
2 1/2 pounds assorted pork and chicken bones

1 teaspoon vinegar (apple cider), optional
1 carrot, (medium), peeled and then cut into three pieces

1. Put all the veggies in a 6-quart IP. Add the bones and water. Add the fish sauce and vinegar. Lock the lid and close the pressure valve. Set to MANUAL HIGH pressure for 30 minutes. If cooking meaty shanks or oxtails, set the cooking time for 50 minutes. You can cook for as long as 2 hours if preferred – the longer it cooks, the better the broth.

2. When the timer beeps, press CANCEL, NPR completely, then QPR and open the lid. Skim the skim off the surface of the broth, strain, and store properly.

Applesauce

Servings|**800 ml**   Prep. Time|**5 minutes**   Cook Time|**25 minutes**
Nutritional Content (per 1 tbsp.): Cal|**7**   Fat|**0g**   Protein|**0g**   Carbs|**2g**

3 pounds preferred variety of apples, unpeeled or peeled, quartered
1 - 2 cinnamon sticks
1/4 cup water (60 ml)

1/4 up to 1/2 teaspoons nutmeg (0.5 up to 1 gram)
Pinch of salt
Stevia to taste

1. Put the cinnamon, nutmeg, water, and apples in your IP. Lock the lid and close the pressure valve. Set to HIGH pressure for 5 minutes. When the timer beeps, press CANCEL, NPR completely, then QPR and open the lid.

2. Remove the cinnamon. Puree the apple mixture using a stick blender till desired texture is achieved. Add salt and stevia to taste.

Rosemary Apple Sauce

Servings | **4**   Prep. Time | **15 minutes**   Cook Time | **5 minutes**
Nutritional Content (per serving): Cal | **127**   Fat | **0.7g**   Protein | **0.6g**   Carbs | **32.9g**

1 long sprig rosemary (fresh)
1/2 cup apple juice or water
3-4 pounds orchard apples (around 10-14 pieces, any variety)

Optional:
4 tablespoons stevia
2 teaspoons apple pie spice

1. Chop the apples into bite-sized chunks. Remove the core and seeds. Remove the peel for a smooth sauce or leave the peel on for a chunky style. If leaving the peel on, chop the apples into small chunks. Put them in your IP. Add the rosemary and water. Add the optional spice and stevia if using.

2. Lock the lid and close the pressure valve. Set to MANUAL HIGH pressure for 5 minutes. When the timer beeps, press CANCEL, NPR completely, then QPR and open the lid. If you prefer a smooth sauce, puree using an immersion blender or in your stand blender.

Roast Garlic

Servings | **1 head**   Prep. Time | **5 minutes**   Cook Time | **8 minutes**
Nutritional Content (per clove): Cal | **24**   Fat | **2.3g**   Protein | **<1g**   Carbs | **1g**

1 cup water   1 whole garlic bulb   Olive oil

1. Carefully slice off the top of the garlic bulb to expose the cloves. Put the IP trivet and pour the water into the inner pot. Put the bulb on the trivet. Lock the lid and close the pressure valve. Set to HIGH pressure for 8 minutes. When the timer beeps, press CANCEL, NPR for 5 up to 7 minutes, then QPR and open the lid.

2. Transfer the garlic bulb to a cookie sheet or baking dish; generously drizzle with the olive oil. Broil for 3 up to 5 minutes or till brown. Use as needed. You can mash it with your sweet potato mash.

HOLIDAY

Sauerkraut Turkey & Sausage for New Year

Servings | **4**   Prep. Time | **10 minutes**   Cook Time | **10 minutes**
Nutritional Content (per serving): Cal | **165**   Fat | **10.5g**   Protein | **9g**   Carbs | **10g**

1 package (5 ounces) turkey sausage, cut into bite-size chunks

1 bag (2 pounds) sauerkraut
1 teaspoon caraway seeds

1. Put everything in your IP. Lock the lid and close the pressure valve. Set tot MANUAL HIGH pressure for 10 minutes. When the timer beeps, press CANCEL, NPR completely, then QPR and open the lid. When the timer beeps, QPR and open the lid. Serve.

Pork & Sauerkraut

Servings | **6**   Prep. Time | **10 minutes**   Cook Time | **30 minutes**
Nutritional Content (per serving): Cal | **403**   Fat | **27.5g**   Protein | **29.7g**   Carbs | **9g**

24 ounces sauerkraut
14 ounces kielbasa, sliced
1/4 teaspoon pepper
1/3 cup water

1/2 teaspoon salt
1 tablespoon stevia
1 tablespoon oil
1 pound country pork ribs

1. Set the IP to SAUTÉ. When hot, add the oil and ribs; season with pepper and salt. Cook till both sides of the meat is brown. Add the sauerkraut and water. Lock the lid and close the pressure valve. Set to MANUAL HIGH pressure for 15 minutes. When the timer beeps, press CANCEL, NPR or QPR and open the lid. Mix the ingredients a bit. Serve as is or with mashed sweet potatoes.

Hot Chocolate Fondue

Servings|4   Prep. Time|**1 minutes**   Cook Time|**10 minutes**
Nutritional Content (per serving): Cal|**198**   Fat|**18g**   Protein|**0g**   Carbs|**0g**

3.5 ounces (100 grams) Swiss Chocolate (70-75% Dark Bittersweet)
3.5 ounces (100 grams) fresh cream or coconut milk
1 teaspoon sugar (optional)
1 teaspoon Amaretto liqueur (optional)

1. Put the IP trivet and pour 2 cups water in the inner pot. In a heatproof container (small), preferably, ceramic, such as a fondue pot, mug, or ramekin, measure and put the chocolate chunks. Add the same amount of fresh cream. If using, add the optional ingredients, or any lectin-free spices or aromatics you prefer. Put the container on the trivet.

2. Lock the lid and close the pressure valve. Set to MANUAL HIGH pressure for 2 minutes. When the timer beeps, QPR and open the lid, guiding the condensation away from the fondue. Remove the container from the pot, immediately stir the contents for 1 minute using a fork; stir till the chocolate breaks and the mixture thickens to a smooth dark brown fondue. Do not add any cold ingredient to the mixture. Serve.

Brussels Sprouts for the Holiday

Servings|6   Prep. Time|**20 minutes**   Cook Time|**10 minutes**
Nutritional Content (per serving): Cal|**140**   Fat|**8.1g**   Protein|**9.9g**   Carbs|**8.4g**

1/4 teaspoon salt
2 tablespoons balsamic reduction
2 tablespoons water
5 slices bacon, chopped
6 cups Brussels sprouts, chopped
Pepper, to taste
1/4 cup soft goat cheese, crumbled, optional

1. Set the IP to SAUTÉ. Add the bacon; sauté till desired crispness is achieved. Add the Brussels sprouts; stir to coat well with the bacon fat. Add the water; season with salt and pepper. Cook for 4 up to 6 minutes or till the Brussels sprouts are crisp, stirring occasionally. Transfer to a serving plate. Drizzle with the balsamic reduction. If using, top with goat cheese.

Make-Ahead Mashed Sweet Potatoes

Servings | 6   Prep. Time | **25 minutes**   Cook Time | **7-11 minutes**
Nutritional Content (per serving): Cal | **438**   Fat | **25g**   Protein | **8.3g**   Carbs | **47.2g**

1 1/2 cup sour cream
1 teaspoon salt
1/4 teaspoon pepper
4 tablespoons butter

5 pounds sweet potatoes
8 ounces cream cheese
Paprika

1. Put the IP steamer basket and pour 1 cup water in the inner pot. Peel the sweet potatoes and wash clean. Slice into halves, and then each half into quarters. Put them in the basket. Lock the lid and close the pressure valve. Set to MANUAL HIGH pressure for 7 up to 9 minutes for fresh or for 9 up to 11 minutes for frozen sweet potatoes.

2. When the timer beeps, press CANCEL, NPR completely, then QPR and open the lid. Remove the potatoes from the pot. Press them through a potato ricer. With your electric mixer, beat the diced sweet potatoes with the pepper, salt, cream cheese, and sour cream till mixed well and creamy. Spread the mash into a 9-inch square baking dish. Serve. If not serving right away, cover the dish with foil and refrigerate for 3 days maximum. To serve, dot the frozen mash with butter slices and sprinkle with paprika; bake in a preheated 350F oven f0r 30 minutes.

Pork Roast & Sauerkraut w/ Hotdog & Kielbasa

Servings | 4-6   Prep. Time | **20 minutes**   Cook Time | **45 minutes**
Nutritional Content (per serving): Cal | **1075**   Fat | **70.9g**   Protein | **86.9g**   Carbs | **18.8g**

1 cup water
1 pound beef hot dogs, optional
1/2 pound beef kielbasa, optional
2 onions, (large), chopped or sliced
2 tablespoons coconut oil, butter, or ghee

2-3 pound (fat-marbled shoulder) pork roast
3 cloves garlic, peeled & sliced
4-6 cups sauerkraut, divided
Black pepper (fresh ground)
Sea or real salt

1. Generously season your pork with pepper and salt. Preheat a skillet/pan (large) over high flame/heat till smoking. Add the coconut oil. Add the pork; cook till all the sides, including the edges, are brown. Remove the pork from the pot.

2. Set a trivet in your IP. Put the pork on the trivet. Add the water, garlic, and onion; generously season with pepper and salt. Lock the lid and close the pressure valve. Set to MANUAL HIGH pressure for 35 minutes. When the timer beeps, press CANCEL, NPR completely, then QPR and open the lid.

3. Add 1/2 of the sauerkraut, reserving the rest for serving to get the benefits of the fermented good bacteria. Lock the lid and close the pressure valve. Set to MANUAL HIGH pressure for 5 minutes if your pork is tender. If the meat is still a bit tough, set the cooking time for 15 minutes.

4. When the timer beeps, QPR and open the lid. Add the hot dogs and kielbasa. Lock the lid and close the pressure valve. Set to MANUAL HIGH pressure for 5 minutes – do not cook longer or your hotdogs will crumble. When the timer beeps, QPR and open the lid. Let rest to cool slightly. Serve with the reserved uncooked sauerkraut, and with mashed sweet potatoes if desired.

Sweet Potato Casserole

Servings|4-5   Prep. Time|20 minutes   Cook Time|10 minutes
Nutritional Content (per serving): Cal|**838**   Fat|**43g**   Protein|**14.5g**   Carbs|**112.5g**

Sweet potatoes:
1 cup water
1 egg, pastured
1 teaspoon cinnamon
1/2 teaspoon nutmeg
1/3 cup coconut palm sugar
1/4 cup coconut milk
1/4 teaspoon allspice
1/4 teaspoon sea salt
2 tablespoons coconut or cassava flour
3 pounds sweet potatoes, scrubbed clean

Topping:
1 teaspoon cinnamon
1/2 cup almond flour
1/2 cup walnuts, coarsely ground, soaked & dehydrated
1/4 cup coconut palm sugar
1/4 cup pecans, coarsely ground, soaked & dehydrated
1/4 cup shredded coconut (unsweetened)
1/4 teaspoon sea salt
5 tablespoons salted butter

Equipment:
1 3/4-quart glass Pyrex bowl

1. Sweet potatoes: Prick the potatoes all over using a fork. Put the IP trivet and pour 1 cup water in the inner pot. Put the potatoes on the trivet. Lock the lid and close the pressure valve. Set to MANUAL HIGH pressure for 20 minutes. Meanwhile, prepare the topping.

2. Topping: Put all the ingredients in a mixing bowl (medium). Using a pastry cutter, cut the butter with the rest of the ingredients till the mixture resembles a gravel that slightly damp.

3. To assemble: When the timer beeps, QPR and open the lid. Remove the potatoes from the pot; leave the water and trivet in the IP. Add enough water to reach the 1 cup level.

4. Carefully peel the potatoes. Put the peeled potatoes in the glass bowl. Add the rest of the sweet potato ingredients; mix with a spoon till everything is evenly combined. Evenly spread the topping on top of the mash. Carefully put the bowl on the trivet.

5. Lock the lid and close the pressure valve. Set to MANUAL HIGH pressure for 10 minutes. When the timer beeps, QPR and open the lid. Remove the bowl from the pot. If desired, broil the casserole for 2 up to 3 minutes or till the topping is crisped.

Parsnips & Caramelized Onions

Servings|4   Prep. Time|**10 minutes**   Cook Time|**30 minutes**
Nutritional Content (per serving): Cal|**355**   Fat|**14.2g**   Protein|**5.6g**   Carbs|**54.3g**

1 1/2 cups beef broth, or more as needed
1 whole sprig thyme
1 yellow onion, (medium), thinly sliced
1/2 teaspoon sea salt
1/4 cup coconut oil, divided
2 1/2 pounds parsnips, peeled & cut into 1/3-inch pieces

1. Set the IP to SAUTÉ. Add 3 tablespoons oil. when hot, add the parsnips; stir to coat. Season with salt; cook for 12 up to 15 minutes or till all the sides are caramelized and brown. Add the broth the thyme. Lock the lid and close the pressure valve. Set to MANUAL HIGH pressure for 3 minutes. When the timer beeps, QPR and open the lid.

2. Transfer the parsnip mixture to a blender, preferably high-powered; blend for 45 up to 60 minutes or till smooth. Add 1 tablespoon of broth at a time if the mixture is too thick.

3. Put the rest of the coconut oil in the IP. Set to SAUTÉ. When hot, add the onion; toss to coat with the oil. Sauté for 10 up to 12 minutes or till tender and golden brown. Add the coconut aminos to deepen the taste. Turn off the IP. Divide the parsnips between serving bowls; top each with caramelized onion and garnish with thyme if desired.

Make-Ahead 10-Minute Gravy

Servings|**6 1/2 cups**   Prep. Time|**5 minutes**   Cook Time|**15 minutes**
Nutritional Content (per 1/2 cup): Cal|**314**   Fat|**9.4g**   Protein|**52g**   Carbs|**2.4g**

5 ounces mushrooms
2 pieces bacon, uncooked
2 onions (large), peeled & sliced into halves
1/4 cup bacon fat or butter
1/2 & 1/4 teaspoon black/white pepper, divided
1 whole chicken (raw)
1 teaspoon thyme
1 teaspoon sage
1 teaspoon onion powder
1 ounce dried mushrooms
1 cup bone broth
1 & 1/4 teaspoon sea salt, divided

1. Put the ingredients in the pot following this order: 1 cup of broth, mushrooms (dried), onion, mushrooms (fresh), bacon, bacon fat/butter, sage, thyme, and 1/2 teaspoon of salt, and 1/4 teaspoon of pepper. Place the chicken on top; season the meat with 1/2 teaspoon of salt and 1/4 teaspoon of pepper. Lock the lid and close the pressure valve. Set to POULTRY HIGH pressure for 15 minutes. When the timer beeps, press CANCEL, NPR for 15 minutes, then QPR and open the lid.

2. Transfer the chicken to a plate (large) or chopping board; let cool enough to handle. Remove the skin from the meat; set aside. Save the meat for recipes needing chicken.

3. With a slotted spoon, transfer the solids from the pot into a blender (high-powered). Scoop 3 cups of cooking liquid into the blender. Save leftover cooking liquid to thin the gravy as needed. Add the chicken skin, remaining pepper and salt, and onion powder.

4. Puree for 50 up to 60 seconds on medium-high power/speed or till the gravy is very smooth. Store properly. When ready to serve, pour the gravy into a saucepan and heat gently. Add cooking liquid to thin as needed.

Beet Borscht

Servings|6   Prep. Time|**20 minutes**   Cook Time|**52 minutes**
Nutritional Content (per serving): Cal|**159**   Fat|**3.2g**   Protein|**6.1g**   Carbs|**30.33g**

8 cups diced or 3 beets (large), peeled,
6 cups stock (beef, chicken, or vegetable)
3 cups cabbage, shredded
2 cloves garlic (large), diced
1/4 cup dill (fresh), chopped
1/4 cup coconut yogurt or sour cream, optional

1/2 tablespoon thyme
1/2 cup (3 stalks) celery, diced
1/2 cup (2 carrots), (large), diced
1 tablespoon salt
1 onion, (medium), diced
Bay leaf
Ice bath

1. Put the IP trivet and pour 1 cup water in the inner pot. Put the beets on the trivet. Lock the lid and close the pressure valve. Set to STEAM for 7 minutes. When the timer beeps, QPR and open the lid. Immediately put the beets in the ice bath – the skins will slip right off them. Dice the beets.

2. Remove the trivet and pour out the cooking water from the inner pot. Wipe it dry and add broth. Put the beets in the instant pot. Add the rest of the ingredients. Lock the lid and close the pressure valve. Set to SOUP for 45 minutes. When the timer beeps, press CANCEL, NPR completely, then QPR and open the lid. Scoop into serving bowls; top each with 1 dollop coconut yogurt or sour cream and garnish with dill.

SLOW COOKED

Slow-Cooked Kielbasa Kapusta

Servings|6   Prep. Time|**10 minutes**   Cook Time|**6-7 hours**
Nutritional Content (per serving): Cal|**281**   Fat|**20g**   Protein|**16g**   Carbs|**11g**

1 coil of favorite kielbasa (garlic flavored), chopped into chunks
1 white onion, sliced
1/2 head green cabbage, chopped
32 ounces sauerkraut (jarred), rinsed with water

1. Mix all of the ingredients in your IP. Set to SLOW COOK LOW for 6 up to 7 hours, occasionally stirring. Serve.

Slow Cooked Chicken w/ Sweet Potatoes & Broccoli

Servings|6   Prep. Time|**20 minutes**   Cook Time|**5 hours, 5 minutes**
Nutritional Content (per serving): Cal|**645**   Fat|**37g**   Protein|**41g**   Carbs|**38.2g**

1 1/2 tablespoons olive oil
1 teaspoon onion powder
1 teaspoon thyme (dried), or 1 tablespoon fresh, minced
1/4 cup chicken broth
16 ounces broccoli florets (packed frozen)
2 1/2 pounds sweet potatoes, peeled & diced into 1 1/4-inch chunks
2 packed teaspoons stevia
2 teaspoons paprika
3/4 teaspoon rosemary (dried) or 2 1/2 teaspoon fresh, minced
4 cloves garlic (1 1/2 tablespoon), minced
6 large chicken thighs (bone-in & skin-on), trimmed
Salt & black pepper (fresh ground)

1. Grease your IP with nonstick spray (lectin-free). In an even layer, put the potatoes in the pot. Add the broth; sprinkle with 1/2 of the garlic and season with pepper and salt.

2. In a bowl (small), whisk the rosemary, thyme, onion powder, stevia, and paprika. Sprinkle 1/2 of the mixture evenly over the potatoes in the pot; save the remaining mixture.

3. Heat the oil in a pot (large) set over medium-high heat. Dab the skin side of the chicken with paper towels to dry and season both sides with pepper and salt. With the skin-side down, put the chicken in the pot; sear for 4 minutes or till golden. Transfer to the IP on top of the potato layer. Repeat the process with the remaining 3 pieces of chicken.

4. Season the chicken with the reserved spice mixture. Cook for 4 1/2 up to 5 hours on LOW. During the last (30) minutes of cooking time, add the broccoli in the pot; season with salt. Finish

cooking. Transfer to a serving dish. Drizzle with a couple of cooking juices from the fat. If desired, skim the fat off the cooking juices first.

Slow-Cooked Tender Pot Roast & Holy Grail Gravy

Servings|4-8   Prep. Time|**15 minutes**   Cook Time|**6-8 hours**
Nutritional Content (per serving): Cal|**296**   Fat|**8.5g**   Protein|**43.2g**   Carbs|**9.6g**

1 bay leaf (whole)
1 onion (chopped)
1/4 cup broth or water
2 (whole) branches rosemary (fresh)
2 stalks celery, thickly sliced
2-4 garlic cloves (whole)

2-4 pounds chuck roast (bone-out or bone-in)
4 carrots, chopped into chunks
Black pepper (fresh ground), optional
Sea salt

1. Put all the vegetables and herbs in your IP. Add 1/4 cup of broth. Season all the sides of the roast with pepper and salt. Put it on top of the veggies. Lock the lid and close the pressure valve. Set to SLOW COOK NORMAL mode for 6 up to 8 hours. When the timer beeps, QPR and open the lid. The meat is done when it is easily shredded with a fork.

2. Transfer the pork to a plate. Remove the rosemary and bay leaf; discard them. Transfer the cooking liquid to a blender. Add 1/2 of the cooked veggies; puree till smooth. Add more veggies to thicken and strengthen the flavor of the gravy as needed. Season with pepper and salt to taste. Serve the roast with the gravy, and with mashed garlic cauliflower.

Slow Cooked Roast Pork w/ Apple-Onion Gravy

Servings|8-10   Prep. Time|**15 minutes**   Cook Time|**8-10 hours**
Nutritional Content (per serving): Cal|**576**   Fat|**26g**   Protein|**68g**   Carbs|**15g**

4-5 pounds pork roast (pork shoulder or Boston butt)
4 apples (medium)
2 teaspoons thyme (dried)
2 teaspoons sea salt
2 teaspoons rosemary (dried)

2 teaspoons black pepper (fresh ground) (optional)
2 tablespoons olive oil (extra-virgin)
2 cloves garlic (pressed)
1/4 cup water
1 onion (large)

1. Peel the apples and remove the cores; slice them into wedges. Scatter them in the bottom of your IP. Peel the onion and slice them into halves; slice thinly. Scatter on top of the apples. Add 1/4 cup water.

2. Mix the spices, garlic, and olive oil in a bowl (small). Rub all the sides of the roast with the spice mixture. With the fatty-side up, put the meat on top of the apple and onion mixture. Lock the lid and close the pressure valve. Set to SLOW COOK NORMAL mode for 8 up to 10 hours or

till you can easily shred the meat with a fork. When the timer beeps, QPR and open the lid. Transfer the roast to a plate.

3. Puree the contents of the pot using a stick blender or a stand blender. Season with salt as needed. Serve the pork topped with the gravy.

Slow-Cooked Nomato Chili

Servings|6   Prep. Time|15-20 minutes   Cook Time| 8 hours
Nutritional Content (per serving): Cal|410   Fat|18g   Protein|45g   Carbs|16g

1 tablespoon oregano (dried)
1 teaspoon onion powder
1 teaspoon thyme (dried)
1/2 rutabaga (medium), peeled & diced
1/2 teaspoon garlic powder
1/2 teaspoon ginger (ground)
1/4 teaspoon cinnamon
1/4 teaspoon ground cloves
2 beets (medium), peeled & grated

2 onions (medium), chopped
2 pounds ground beef (grass-fed)
2 tablespoon tapioca flour, to thicken, optional
3 carrots (large), peeled & diced
3 cups bone broth
4 cloves garlic, crushed
Homemade lectin-free guacamole to serve
Sea salt to taste

1. Except for the tapioca starch, put all the ingredients in the IP. Lock the lid and close the pressure valve. Set to SLOW COOK NORMAL mode for 8 hours. When the timer beeps, QPR and open the lid. Season as needed. Thicken with tapioca flour slurry as needed. Serve. Top each serving with guacamole.

Slow-Cooked Beef Short Ribs & Mushrooms

Servings|8   Prep. Time|5 minutes   Cook Time|8 hours, 20 minutes
Nutritional Content (per serving): Cal|552   Fat|22.2g   Protein|52g   Carbs|44g

1 cup beef broth
1 tablespoon ginger (fresh), grated
1/2 tablespoon coconut oil
1/2 teaspoon fish sauce
1/2 teaspoon salt plus more to taste
2 cloves garlic, minced

2 packages (8 ounces) whole (baby Bella and cremini) mushrooms
3 tablespoons coconut aminos
4 pounds beef short ribs (grass-fed)
Pepper to taste

1. Put the mushrooms in a colander; shake to remove the debris and silt. Rinse quickly and then wipe them with a soft cloth. Put the mushrooms in the IP. Add the garlic and ginger; gently mix to combine.

2. Heat your pan/skillet on the stovetop over medium-high flame/heat. Add the coconut oil and melt. In batches, add the ribs and cook till all the sides are brown, seasoning with pepper and salt in the process. Add the browned meat to the IP. Save the drippings in the pan/skillet; remove it from the heat. Add the broth, fish sauce, and coconut aminos to the pan/skillet. Over low heat; gently cook, whisking to mix and scraping the browned bits off. Transfer the liquid mixture to the IP. Set to SLOW COOK NORMAL mode for 8 hours or till the meat is fall-off-the-bone tender. When the timer beeps, QPR and open the lid.

3. Transfer the ribs to a serving dish; tent with foil to keep warm. Pour all the contents of the pot to a saucepan. Add 1/2 teaspoon of salt or to taste as needed. Bring the sauce to a boil on high flame/heat and then reduce to a simmer. Cook for 10 minutes or till the flavor is concentrated to your liking. Serve the ribs with the mushrooms on the side. Drizzle the meat with some of the sauce.

Slow-Cooked Rosemary-Lemon Lamb

Servings|**8-10**   Prep. Time|**5 minutes**   Cook Time|**6-8 hours**
Nutritional Content (per serving): Cal|**310**   Fat|**12.1g**   Protein|**46g**   Carbs|**1.2g**

1 boneless (around 4 - 5 pounds) leg lamb
1 lemon, sliced
2 cups water
2 sprigs rosemary

2 tablespoon Dijon mustard or 4 cloves garlic, chopped
Pepper & salt

1. Put the lemon slices and the sprigs of rosemary in the bottom of your IP. Put the lamb on top of lemon and rosemary. Generously with salt and pepper. Add the mustard or cloves on top of the lamb. Add the water. Lock the lid and close the pressure valve. Set to SLOW COOK NORMAL mode for 6 up to 8 hours. When the timer beeps, QPR and open the lid. Serve with mashed sweet potatoes.

SNACKS & DESSERTS

Italian Turkey-Stuffed Sweet Potatoes

Servings|2   Prep. Time|15 minutes   Cook Time|80-90 minutes
Nutritional Content (per serving): Cal|0   Fat|18g   Protein|32g   Carbs|42g

1 1/2 cups water
1/2 cup sweet yellow onion, sliced
2 sweet potatoes, choose ones with very similar size
2 tablespoons avocado oil
3/4 pound ground Italian turkey or chicken
4 cups spinach, optional

Garnish (optional):
Parsley
Parmesan cheese

1. Put the IP trivet and pour the water into the inner pot. Put the potatoes on the trivet. Set the IP to STEAM for 15 – 20 minutes for 6-inch, 25-30 for 8-inch, 35-40 for 10-inch, or for 45-50 for 12-inch circumference. When the timer beeps, QPR and open the lid.

2. Take the potatoes out from the IP. Drain the inner pot and return to the housing. Add the oil and onions. Set to SAUTE. Cook till the onions are soft and translucent. Add the meat; sauté till cooked through, setting the IP to SAUTE LESS mode once the meat stars sticking to the pot. Add the spinach is using; sauté till wilted.

3. Slice the potatoes lengthwise into halves. Mush the center down using a fork, making a well for meat filling. Fill each with the meat mixture. Garnish with parsley and cheese. Serve.

Swedish Meatballs & Mushrooms Gravy

Servings|6-8   Prep. Time|15 minutes   Cook Time|40 minutes
Nutritional Content (per serving): Cal|278   Fat|12.2g   Protein|37g   Carbs|4g

1 onion (large), chopped
1 pound/ 450 grams ground pork
1 pound/450 grams ground beef
1 teaspoon sage (dried)
1/2 cup coconut milk, bone broth, or water
1/2 teaspoon mace (ground)

1/2 teaspoon sea salt
1/4 cup parsley (fresh), minced, divided
2 cups (cremini/button) mushrooms, sliced
2 tablespoons onion (dried), chopped
3 tablespoons coconut aminos

1. In a bowl, mix the pork, beef, salt, mace, dried onion, and 3 tablespoons parsley. Form the mixture into 1-inch meatballs. Put the mushrooms, fresh onion, coconut milk/broth/water, and coconut aminos in your IP. Add the meatballs. Lock the lid and close the pressure valve. Set to MEAT/STEW for 35 minutes. When the timer beeps, QPR and open the lid.

2. Gently transfer the meatballs with a slotted spoon to a serving dish. Using a stick blender or a high-powered blender, puree the remaining contents of the pot. Adding coconut milk/broth/water as needed to thin. Pour the gravy over the meatballs; garnish with the remaining parsley.

NOTES: Serve as an appetizer, main course, over cauliflower rice, or sautéed lectin-free veggies.

Bacon Cheesy Asparagus

Servings|2   Prep. Time|2 minutes   Cook Time|3 minutes
Nutritional Content (per serving): Cal|331   Fat|24.3g   Protein|23.1g   Carbs|5.7g

160 ml, for the IP
250 grams asparagus
4 slices back bacon

50 grams soft cheese, butter, or coconut oil
Pepper & salt, to taste

1. Put the IP trivet and pour the water into the inner pot. Chop off the tough ends of the asparagus. Smoother each pear with soft cheese and then wrap each with 1 slice of bacon. Put them on the trivet.

2. Lock the lid and close the pressure valve. Set to STEAM for 3 minutes. When the timer beeps, press CANCEL, NPR completely, then QPR and open the lid. Transfer the asparagus to a serving dish. Serve.

Spinach & Garlic Beef Meatballs

Servings|4-6   Prep. Time|20 minutes   Cook Time|20 minutes
Nutritional Content (per serving): Cal|287   Fat|13g   Protein|31.7g   Carbs|10g

1 cup frozen/fresh spinach, chopped
1 pound ground beef (grass-fed)
1/4 cup garlic, minced
4 carrots (large), chopped to 1/2-inch chunks

Preferred bone broth
Real salt & pepper to taste

1. Put the carrots and add enough broth to cover them. In a bowl (large), mix the beef, pepper, salt, garlic, and spinach till well mixed, mashing in the process. Roll the meat mixture int0 golfball-sized pieces. Put the meatballs on top of the carrots. Lock the lid and close the pressure valve. Set to MANUAL for 20 minutes. When the timer beeps, QPR and open the lid. Serve as a soup or serve the meatballs and carrots in a serving dish and the broth in a bowl.

Potato Skins w/ Bacon & Guacamole

Servings | **5**   Prep. Time | **10 minutes**   Cook Time | **1 hour**
Nutritional Content (per serving): Cal | **331**   Fat | **26.7g**   Protein | **6g**   Carbs | **20g**

2-3 tablespoons ghee/butter, melted
5 small (around 3-inch long) sweet potatoes
Black pepper (fresh ground
Garlic powder
Sea salt

Guacamole:
2 ripe avocados, halved, seeded, & flesh scooped out
Juice of 1/2 lemon
Sea salt

Toppings
5 slices bacon, sliced into 1/2-inch strips
4 green onions, sliced thin

1. Potato skins: Pierce the potatoes all over with a fork. Put the IP trivet and pour 1 cup water in the inner pot. Put the potatoes on the trivet. Lock the lid and close the pressure valve. Set to MANUAL HIGH pressure for 22 minutes. When the timer beeps, press CANCEL, NPR for 10 minutes, then QPR and open the lid. Remove the potatoes from the pot and let cool for 10 minutes or till cool enough to handle.

2. In skillet (small/medium) set over medium flame/heat. Add the bacon; cook till crisp and the fat is rendered. Transfer to a plate lined with paper towel to drain excess grease.

3. In a bowl (large), mix the avocados, salt, garlic powder, and lemon juice. Mash using a potato masher till smooth.

4. Set your oven to broil. Slice the cooked potato lengthwise into halves. Scoop the flesh out, leaving 1/4-inch of flesh intact. Reserve the potato flesh for other uses. With a pastry brush, brush the outside of the potatoes with ghee; generously season with pepper and salt. Turn them over and brush the insides with ghee; season with pepper and salt. With the skin-side down, put the potato halves on a sheet pan. Broil for 3 up to 6 minutes or till the skin starts t crisp and brown. Transfer the potato skins to a serving dish. Spoon dollops of guacamole in the potato skins; garnish with lots of bacon and green onions.

Baked Apples

Servings|6   Prep. Time|**5 minutes**   Cook Time|**8 minutes**
Nutritional Content (per serving): Cal|**120**   Fat|**0.4g**   Protein|**0.6g**   Carbs|**60g**

1 cup apple juice or red wine
1/2 cup stevia

2 tablespoons cinnamon
6 gala or preferred variety apples

1. Wash the apples clean and core them. Put them in your IP. Add the apple juice/red wine. Sprinkle the stevia and cinnamon over them. Lock the lid and close the pressure valve. Set to MANUAL HIGH pressure for 8 minutes. When the timer beeps, press CANCEL, NPR completely or QPR and open the lid. Put the apples into individual serving bowls. Drizzle each with some of the cooking juices.

Wine "Braised" Figs on Yogurt Crème

Servings|8   Prep. Time|**5 minutes**   Cook Time|**8 minutes**
Nutritional Content (per serving): Cal|**273**   Fat|**7g**   Protein|**16g**   Carbs|**42g**

Poached figs:
1 cup red wine (good quality)
1 pound figs (500 grams)
1/2 cup of pine nuts (untoasted or toasted)
1/2 cup stevia

Yogurt crème:
1 kilogram (2 pounds) yogurt (plain)

Equipment:
Fine mesh strainer

1. Yogurt crème: Pour the yogurt in the strainer set over a bowl. Spread it, but do not press. Place in the coldest part of your refrigerator to drain for 4 hours. Do not drain longer, like 8 hours, or you will get crumbly yogurt cheese and not crème.

2. Pine nuts: If you prefer toasted pine nuts, put them in the bottom of your IP. Set the IP to SAUTÉ NORMAL mode. Cook till they are nicely toasted, but not burnt, stirring often. Transfer them to a dish to continue cooking with the residual heat.

3. Poached figs: Put the IP trivet and pour the wine in the inner pot. In upright position, put the figs on the trivet. Lock the lid and close the pressure valve. Set the IP to HIGH pressure. Wait till the pot reaches pressure. Once pressure is achieved, reduce the pressure to LOW and set the timer to 3 minutes. When the timer beeps, QPR and open the lid.

4. Remove the figs from the pot. Set the IP to SAUTÉ. Add the stevia. Cook till the wine is reduced by 1/2 or till you can briefly see the bottom of the pot when you drag a spoon across it.

5. To assemble: Scoop a dollop of yogurt crème on a serving dish. Artfully arrange the figs on top. Drizzle with a bit of wine syrup and then sprinkle with the nuts. You can serve this warm or chilled if making ahead of time.

Chorizo Custard

Servings|6   Prep. Time|**19 minutes**   Cook Time|**6 minutes**
Nutritional Content (per serving): Cal|**279**   Fat|**26.7g**   Protein|**8.1g**   Carbs|**2.1g**

1 1/2 cups water
1/2 cup chorizo, cooked
2 cups heavy cream
6 egg yolks (medium)
Pinch sea salt

Equipment:
Aluminum foil
6 pieces 1/2-cup ramekins

1. Put the IP trivet and pour the water into the inner pot. In a mixing bowl, whisk the salt, yolks, and cream till well mixed. Divide the chorizo between the ramekins. Fill each ramekin 3/4 full with the cream mixture. Cover them with foil. Stack the ramekins on the trivet, placing the extra pieces on top of the first layer. Lock the lid and close the pressure valve. Set to MANUAL HIGH pressure for 6 minutes. When the timer beeps, press CANCEL, NPR for 10 minutes, then QPR and open the lid. Carefully remove the ramekins from the pot. Serve hot.

NOTES: Refrigerate leftovers. To reheat, Put the IP trivet and pour 1 1/2 cups water in the inner pot. Lock the lid and close the pressure valve. Set to MANUAL HIGH pressure for 3 minutes. When the timer beeps, QPR and open the lid.

Vanilla Bean Cheesecake

Servings|8   Prep. Time|**10 minutes**   Cook Time|**20 minutes**
Nutritional Content (per serving): Cal|**217**   Fat|**20.9g**   Protein|**5.7g**   Carbs|**1.7g**

1 teaspoon vanilla extract (organic)
1 vanilla bean, scraped seeds only
1/2cup stevia
16 ounces cream cheese
2 eggs (large)

Equipment:
1 piece 7-inch spring-form pan

1. Put all of the ingredients; blend till very smooth. Pour the mixture into the pan; tightly cover with foil. Put the IP trivet and pour 2 cups water in the inner pot. Put the pan in the trivet. Lock the lid and close the pressure valve. Set to MANUAL HIGH pressure for 20 minutes. When the timer beeps, press CANCEL, NPR completely, then QPR and open the lid. Let cool for 30 up to 60 minutes to room temperature. Transfer in your refrigerator and chill for at least 1 hour before serving.

Turkey Meatballs

Servings|**16**   Prep. Time|**15 minutes**   Cook Time|**2-3 minutes per batch**
Nutritional Content (per ball): Cal|**162**   Fat|**15g**   Protein|**6g**   Carbs|**0.38g**

1 egg
1 pound ground turkey
1/2 teaspoon sea salt
1/4 teaspoon garlic powder
1/4 teaspoon oregano

1/4 teaspoon rosemary
1/4 teaspoon thyme
1/8 cup olive oil (extra-virgin)
Pepper

1. Preheat your IP by setting it to SAUTE mode. In a mixing bowl, except for the oil, mix the rest of the ingredients – do not overmix. Form the meat mixture into 2 tablespoons worth of meatballs, making 16 pieces. Sprinkle with pepper; set aside.

2. Add the oil to the hot IP. Add the meatballs, cook each side for 2 up to 3 minutes or till all the sides are brown. Transfer to a plate lined with paper towels to absorb excess grease. Toss with lectin-free BBQ sauce. Serve.

Broccoli-Cauliflower Sausage Tots

Servings | **20-24**　　Prep. Time | **25-30 minutes**　　Cook Time | **60 minutes**
Nutritional Content (per tot): Cal | **21**　　Fat | **1.3g**　　Protein | **1.5g**　　Carbs | **1.27g**

1 cup water, for the IP
1 egg (large)
1 shallot, finely minced
1 teaspoon oregano (dried)

1/2 teaspoon sea salt
1/4 pound sausage (mild Italian)
2 cups broccoli florets (fresh)
2 cups cauliflower florets (fresh)

1. Put the IP trivet and pour the water into the inner pot. Put the cauliflower and broccoli on the trivet. Lock the lid and close the pressure valve. Set to MANUAL for 2 minutes. When the timer beeps, QPR and open the lid.

2. Preheat your oven to 400F. Line a sheet pan with parchment paper. Transfer the cauliflower and broccoli to your blender or food processor. Pulse for 5 or 6 times till smooth. Transfer the mixture to a bowl (medium). Add the sausage, shallot, egg, salt, and oregano; mix till well combined. Form the mixture into 20 tots. Put them in the prepared sheet pan. Bake for 35 minutes. Serve warm.

Interested in becoming a master chef? ;)

If you liked the recipes in this book, then you might be interested in the following books.

Dash Slow Cooker Cookbook

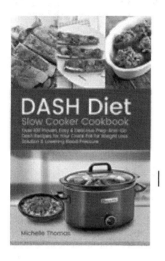

Anti-Inflammatory Diet Instant Pot Cookbook

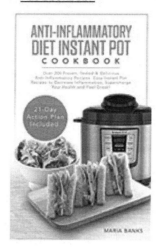

Prediabetes Cookbook

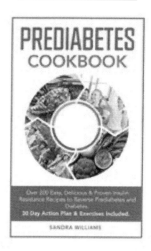

Mind Diet Cookbook

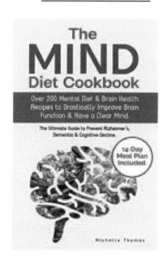

Dash Cookbook

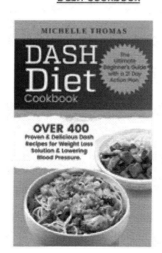

Keto Fat Bombs Cookbook

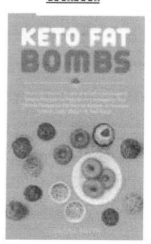

Type 2 Diabetes Cookbook

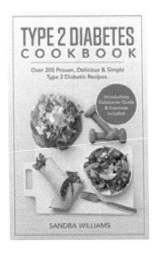

PCOS Cookbook

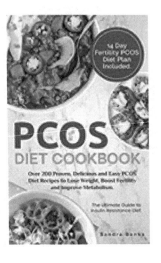

Lectin Free Diet Cookbook

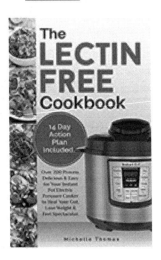

Dukan Diet Cookbook

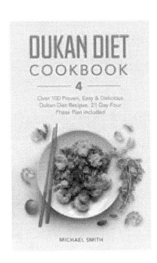

Mini Instant Pot Cookbook

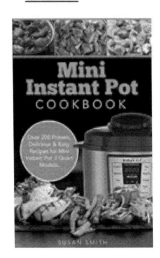

We sincerely hope you enjoyed the recipes.

If you feel like we could improve the cookbook please email us at info@limitlessrecipes.com and we'll make sure to get back to you.

We have a big passion for cooking and we love writing cookbooks but quite often it's pretty hard to compete with all the big publishing companies out there. Reviews really help us and we would appreciate it if you could take a minute and leave a review of the book.

If you could take one minute to leave a review, we would really appreciate that.

You can also leave a review by following these 3 steps:

1. Go to the product page
2. Scroll down and on the left side click 'Write customer review'
3. Write a review and click 'Submit'

Thank you, it really means a lot. Who's amazing? You are!

Final Words

Thank you again for downloading this book!

I hope this book was able to help you start a wonderful adventure in the kitchen making delicious and healthy home-cooked Lectin Free meals with your Instant Pot. I also hope you enjoyed reading and trying out all the wonderful dishes.

If you learned a great value about Lectin Free food and loved the recipes, please leave a review. It will only take a minute of your time and I will greatly appreciate your thoughts!

Thank you in advance for your feedback! Happy Lectin Free cooking!

Made in the USA
Middletown, DE
07 April 2019